SOMNOLOGY

LEARN
SLEEP MEDICINE
IN ONE WEEKEND

T. Lee-Chiong MD
Somnologist

Preface

Carpe noctem.

Teofilo Lee-Chiong MD
Somnologist
Division of Sleep Medicine
National Jewish Health
University of Colorado Denver
School of Medicine
Denver, Colorado

To Grace Zamudio and Zoe Lee-Chiong.

Instructions on Using This Book

1. Although it will take only one weekend to read this book, it is highly recommended that you read it several times over the course of the year. Do not read this book for the first time on the evening before the Sleep Medicine Board.
2. It is assumed that you already know whatever this book doesn't cover about Sleep Medicine.
3. Reconsider your options; take the test only if you are ready to pass (or willing to fail).

There are other less difficult specialties, such as Pulmonary Medicine, Neurology, Psychiatry, and Otolaryngology.

4. It is not the responsibility of the author if you happen to fail the Board; place the blame instead on your Sleep Medicine fellowship program director.
5. Lastly, kindly do not pass this book on to your friends – let them buy their own.

Abbreviations

AC	Alternating current
ACTH	Adrenocorticotropic hormone
ADHD	Attention deficit hyperactivity disorder
AHI	Apnea hypopnea index
AI	Apnea index
AIDS	Acquired immunodeficiency syndrome
ALTE	Apparent life-threatening event
ANS	Autonomic nervous system
APAP	Auto-titrating positive airway pressure
ASPD	Advanced sleep phase disorder
ASV	Adaptive servo ventilation
BMI	Body mass index
BP	Blood pressure
BPAP	Bi-level positive airway pressure
BZ	Benzodiazepine
CAD	Coronary artery disease
CBT	Cognitive behavioral therapy
CCAHS	Congenital central alveolar hypoventilation syndrome
CHF	Congestive heart failure
CNS	Central nervous system
CO	Cardiac output
CO_2	Carbon dioxide
COPD	Chronic obstructive pulmonary disease
CPAP	Continuous positive airway pressure
CRH	Corticotropin-releasing hormone
CRP	C-reactive protein
CSA	Central sleep apnea
CSF	Cerebrospinal fluid
CSR	Cheyne Stokes respiration
CT	Computed tomography
CTmax	Maximum core body temperature
CTmin	Minimum core body temperature
DC	Direct current
DLMO	Dim light melatonin onset
DM	Diabetes mellitus
DSPD	Delayed sleep phase disorder
DZ	Dizygotic
ECG	Electrocardiography
EDS	Excessive daytime sleepiness
EEG	Electroencephalography
EMG	Electromyography
EOG	Electro-oculography
EPAP	Expiratory positive airway pressure
ERV	Expiratory reserve volume
ESRD	End-stage renal disease
ESS	Epworth sleepiness scale
FDA	Food and Drug Administration
FEV_1	Forced expiratory volume in 1 second
FRC	Functional residual capacity
FRD	Free running disorder
FVC	Forced vital capacity
GABA	Gamma-aminobutyric acid
GER	Gastroesophageal reflux

GH	Growth hormone
GHRH	Growth hormone releasing hormone
GI	Gastrointestinal
Hcrt	Hypocretin
HLA	Human leukocyte antigen
HR	Heart rate
HRT	Hormone replacement therapy
Hz	Hertz (cycles per second)
ICAM	Inter-cellular adhesion molecule
ICU	Intensive care unit
IL	Interleukin
IPAP	Inspiratory positive airway pressure
ISWP	Irregular sleep-wake pattern
LDT	Laterodorsal tegmental
LV	Left ventricle
LVEF	Left ventricular ejection fraction
MAOI	Monoamine oxidase inhibitor
MMA	Maxillo-mandibular advancement
MRI	Magnetic resonance imaging
MSLT	Multiple sleep latency test
MWT	Maintenance of wakefulness test
MZ	Monozygotic
N1	NREM stage 1 sleep
N2	NREM stage 2 sleep
N3	NREM stages 3 (and 4) sleep
NBBRA	Non-benzodiazepine benzodiazepine receptor agonist
NREM	Non-rapid eye movement
O_2	Oxygen
OHS	Obesity hypoventilation syndrome
OSA	Obstructive sleep apnea
$PaCO_2$	Partial pressure of arterial carbon dioxide
PaO_2	Partial pressure of arterial oxygen
PAP	Positive airway pressure
P_{CRIT}	Critical closing pressure
PD	Parkinson disease
PET	Positron emission tomography
$PetCO_2$	Partial pressure of end-tidal carbon dioxide
PGO	Ponto-geniculo-occipital
PLMD	Periodic limb movement disorder
PLMI	Periodic limb movement index
PLMS	Periodic limb movements of sleep
PLMW	Periodic limb movements of wakefulness
PPT	Pedunculopontine tegmental
PSG	Polysomnography
$PtcCO_2$	Partial pressure of transcutaneous carbon dioxide
PTSD	Post-traumatic stress disorder
PTT	Pulse transit time
PVC	Premature ventricular contractions
PVR	Pulmonary vascular resistance
QOL	Quality of life
R	Stage REM sleep
RBD	REM sleep behavior disorder
RDI	Respiratory disturbance index
REM	Rapid eye movement sleep
REM SL	Rapid eye movement sleep latency
REMs	Rapid eye movements

RERA	Respiratory effort related arousal
RF	Reticular formation
RIP	Respiratory inductance plethysmography
RLS	Restless legs syndrome
RR	Respiratory rate
RT	Reticular formation
RV	Right ventricle
SaO$_2$	Oxygen saturation
SCN	Suprachiasmatic nucleus
SD	Sleep deprivation
SE	Sleep efficiency
SIDS	Sudden infant death syndrome
SOL	Sleep onset latency
SOREMP	Sleep onset REM period
SPECT	Single photon emission computed tomography
SRBD	Sleep-related breathing disorder
SSRI	Selective serotonin reuptake inhibitor
SUNDS	Sudden unexplained nocturnal death syndrome
SVR	Systemic vascular resistance
SWSD	Shift work sleep disorder.
TCA	Tricyclic antidepressant
TMJ	Temporomandibular joint
TNF	Tumor necrosis factor
TSH	Thyroid stimulating hormone
TST	Total sleep time
TV	Tidal volume
UA	Upper airway
UARS	Upper airway resistance syndrome
UPPP	Uvulopalatopharyngoplasty
VCAM	Vascular cell adhesion molecule
VLPO	Ventrolateral preoptic
V/Q	Ventilation-perfusion
W	Stage Wake
WASO	Wake time after sleep onset

For This Weekend

Sleep: A Very Short Introduction

1. Sleep is a complex reversible state; its principal characteristics include behavioral quiescence and diminished responsiveness to external stimuli compared to the waking state.

2. Sleep is both a function *of* the brain and functions *for* the brain. Sleep is generated and maintained by central neural networks utilizing specific neurotransmitters that are located in specific areas of the brain; these networks are generally redundant and destruction of any particular localized area is unlikely to completely abolish the sleep state.

3. Although a comprehensive theory on the function/s of sleep remains elusive (i.e., sleep may address multiple physiologic needs), it is unquestioned that sleep is central to the development and optimal operation of the brain.

4. A bi-directional relationship exists between the sciences of sleep medicine and that of general medicine, neurology, psychiatry and surgery. Indeed, symptoms of these disorders are modified by, and, more importantly can lead to, sleep disruption. Thus, the science of sleep medicine is truly multi-disciplinary.

It's All in the Brain

General
1. Wake, NREM sleep and REM sleep are each generated and maintained by different neurons and neural networks utilizing specific neurotransmitters.

Neural systems generating wakefulness
1. Ascending reticular formation in the medulla, pons and midbrain (neurotransmitter: glutamate): Afferent pathways project to the thalamus and cerebral cortex.
2. Basal forebrain [PPT and LDT nuclei] (acetylcholine).
3. Hypothalamus (hypocretin).
4. Locus ceruleus (norepinephrine).
5. Tuberomammillary nucleus (histamine).
6. Ventral tegmental area (dopamine).

Two major pathways of the ascending reticular formation
1. Dorsal thalamocortical pathway: RF $\Rightarrow$ thalamus (midline and intralaminar thalamic nuclei) $\Rightarrow$ cerebral cortex.
2. Ventral pathway: RF $\Rightarrow$ posterior hypothalamus and subthalamus $\Rightarrow$ basal forebrain $\Rightarrow$ cerebral cortex.

Neural systems generating NREM sleep
1. VLPO area of hypothalamus (neurotransmitters: GABA and galanin).
2. Basal forebrain (GABA and adenosine).
3. Solitary tract nuclei.
4. Orbitofrontal cortex.
5. Thalamus.
   a. Sleep spindles are generated by reticular thalamic nuclei (GABA).

Neural systems generating REM sleep
1. Caudal mesencephalon and rostral pons (PPT and LDT nuclei).
   a. Reticularis pontis oralis (dorsolateral pons).
2. Nucleus magnocellularis (ventromedial medulla).
3. Ponto-geniculo-occipital (PGO) waves are generated in the pons (dorsolateral) accompanied by activation of the lateral geniculate nucleus and occipital cortex (i.e., P = pons, G = geniculate, and O = occipital).
4. REM sleep is associated with activation of "REM-on" neurons and inhibition of "REM-off" neurons.
   a. "REM-on" neurons: Cholinergic.
   b. "REM-off" neurons: Noradrenergic (locus ceruleus), serotonergic (dorsal raphe) and histaminergic (tuberomammillary nuclei).
5. REM sleep-related muscle atonia is due to inhibitory post-synaptic potentials: Pons (perilocus ceruleus of the pontine tegmentum) $\Rightarrow$ lateral tegmento-reticular tract $\Rightarrow$ medullary magnocellularis neurons $\Rightarrow$ ventrolateral reticulospinal tract $\Rightarrow$ motor neurons of the anterior horn cells of the spinal cord (glycine).

Aminergic vs. cholinergic tone
1. Differences in aminergic and cholinergic tone occur during wake, NREM sleep and REM sleep.
2. Activity of aminergic neurons:
   a. Wake: $\uparrow$.
   b. NREM sleep: $\downarrow$.
   c. REM sleep: $\downarrow$.
3. Activity of cholinergic neurons:
   a. Wake: $\uparrow$.
   b. NREM sleep: $\downarrow$.
   c. REM sleep: $\uparrow$.

Sleep and Wake Neurotransmitters

General
1. Main neurotransmitters involved in the generation of the wake state include:
   a. Acetylcholine.
   b. Dopamine.
   c. Glutamate.
   d. Histamine.
   e. Hypocretin (orexin).
   f. Norepinephrine.
   g. Serotonin.
2. Main neurotransmitters involved in the generation of sleep include:
   a. Acetylcholine (REM sleep).
   b. Adenosine.
   c. GABA.
   d. Glycine.
3. Acetylcholine is the main REM sleep neurotransmitter. GABA is the main NREM neurotransmitter.

Acetylcholine
1. Wake and REM sleep neurotransmitter.
2. Neurons are located primarily in the basal forebrain and PPT/LDT in the brainstem.
3. Responsible for cortical EEG desynchronization during wake and REM sleep. Muscarinic cholinergic receptors in the pontine reticular formation are important in regulating REM sleep.
4. Cholinergic agonists (e.g., physostigmine) decrease REM SL. Anticholinergic drugs (e.g., TCA) decrease REM sleep.

Adenosine
1. Sleep neurotransmitter.
2. Neurons are located primarily in the basal forebrain.
3. Levels progressively increase during prolonged wakefulness (i.e., it is responsible for the homeostatic sleep drive) and decrease during sleep.
4. Adenosine receptor blockers (e.g., caffeine) increase wakefulness.

Dopamine
1. Wake and REM sleep neurotransmitter.
2. Neurons are located primarily in the substantia nigra and ventral tegmental area of the brainstem.
3. Activation of D1 receptors increases wakefulness.
4. Amphetamines enhance dopamine release (wake promotion).
5. D2/D3 dopamine receptor agonists (pramipexole and ropinirole) can cause sedation.

Gamma-aminobutyric acid
1. Sleep neurotransmitter.
2. Main CNS inhibitory neurotransmitter.
3. Neurons are located primarily in the VLPO, thalamus, hypothalamus, basal forebrain and cerebral cortex.
4. Barbiturates, BZ and NBBRAs (e.g., eszopiclone, zaleplon and zolpidem) act via the GABA-A receptor. Gamma-hydroxybutyrate (sodium oxybate) acts via the GABA-B receptor.
5. GABA-A, the major GABA receptor, is a membrane chloride ion channel. It consists of five subunits (often 2 alpha, 2 beta and 1 gamma), each with several subtypes. Binding of BZ agonists to BZ receptors at the alpha-gamma subunit of the GABA complex increases the chloride current at the GABA receptor site.

Glutamate
1. Main CNS excitatory neurotransmitter.

Glycine
1. Main inhibitory neurotransmitter in the spinal cord. Responsible for hyperpolarization (inhibition) of spinal motoneurons that causes REM sleep-related muscle atonia/hypotonia.

Histamine
1. Wake neurotransmitter.
2. Neurons are located primarily in the posterior hypothalamic tuberomammillary nucleus and project to the forebrain. Inhibits the sleep-promoting preoptic area.
3. Histaminergic neurons are inhibited by GABAergic VLPO neurons.
4. First generation histamine-1 receptor blockers cause sedation.

Hypocretin (orexin)
1. Wake neurotransmitter.
2. Neurons are located primarily in the lateral hypothalamic perifornical region.
3. Acts on other CNS centers related to sleep-wake regulation, including the dorsal raphe, basal forebrain, locus ceruleus, tuberomammillary nucleus and spinal cord.
4. Two receptors: Hypocretin-1 and -2.
5. Hypocretin system dysfunction is associated with narcolepsy-cataplexy.
6. Hypocretins are also involved in the regulation of appetite, body temperature and BP.

Immuno-modulators and peptides
1. IL-Iβ, IL-6, TNFα, prostaglandin D2, delta sleep-inducing peptide, vasoactive intestinal peptide, growth hormone-releasing hormone and CRP promote NREM sleep.

Melatonin
1. Produced by the pineal gland during the night. Secretion is inhibited by light exposure. Melatonin receptors are present in the SCN (circadian rhythm regulation) and hypothalamus (thermoregulation).

Norepinephrine
1. Wake neurotransmitter.
2. Neurons are located primarily in the locus ceruleus. Activity of neurons: Wake > NREM > REM.
3. Catecholamine agonists, such as isoproterenol, enhance arousal and wakefulness.

Serotonin
1. Wake neurotransmitter.
2. Neurons are located primarily in the raphe nuclei and thalamus, with projections to the forebrain. Activity of neurons: Wake > NREM > REM.
3. Medications that inhibit serotonin reduce REM sleep. SSRIs can cause insomnia.

In summary, important neurotransmitters and their neurons include:
1. *Acetylcholine - PPT/LDT.*
2. *Adenosine - basal forebrain.*
3. *Dopamine - substantia nigra.*
4. *GABA - VLPO.*
5. *Histamine - tuberomammillary nucleus.*
6. *Hypocretin - lateral hypothalamic perifornical region.*
7. *Melatonin - pineal gland.*
8. *Norepinephrine - locus ceruleus.*
9. *Serotonin - raphe nuclei.*

What Happens during Sleep

In this section
Autonomic nervous system
Respiratory system
Cardiovascular system
Gastrointestinal system
Renal system
Genito-urinary system
Endocrine system
Musculoskeletal system
Pupillary changes
Immunity
Thermoregulation
Metabolism
Dreaming
Summary: what goes up and what goes down during sleep

Autonomic nervous system

1. During NREM sleep compared to wake: ↓ Sympathetic activity and ↑ parasympathetic activity.
2. During REM sleep compared to NREM sleep: ↓ Sympathetic activity and ↑ parasympathetic activity. Transient ↑ in sympathetic activity during phasic REM sleep.
3. In patients with OSA: ↑ Sympathetic activity during both wake and sleep (compared to persons without OSA). Effective PAP therapy reduces this elevation in sympathetic activity.

Respiratory system

1. *Control of respiration*: Both metabolic (i.e., pH, PaO_2, and $PaCO_2$) and behavioral control during wake. Metabolic control only during sleep.
2. *Hypoxic and hypercapnic ventilatory responses*:
   a. ↓ During NREM sleep (compared to wake).
   b. ↓↓ During REM sleep.
   c. Note: There are gender differences in ventilatory responses. Among women, hypoxic ventilatory response is similar during both wake and NREM sleep. A greater reduction in hypoxic ventilatory drive occurs from wake to sleep in men compared to women.
3. *Blood gas parameters*: Compared to wake, ↓ PaO_2 by 2-12 mmHg, ↑ $PaCO_2$ by 2-8 mmHg, and ↓ SaO_2 by 2% during sleep.

4. *UA dilator muscle tone*:
   a. ↓ During NREM sleep (compared to wake).
   b. ↓↓ During REM sleep.
5. *Ventilatory response to added inspiratory resistance*: ↓ During sleep (compared to wake).
6. *Activity of accessory muscles of respiration*:
   a. ↓ During NREM sleep (compared to wake).
   b. ↓↓ During REM sleep.
7. *Tidal volume and minute ventilation*: ↓ During sleep (compared to wake).
8. *Respiratory patterns during sleep*:
   a. N1 sleep: Periodic breathing with episodes of hypopneas and hyperpneas.
   b. N3 sleep: Stable and regular frequency and amplitude of respiration.
   c. REM sleep: Irregular pattern of respiration (variable RR and TV). Central apneas or periodic breathing may occur during phasic REM sleep.
9. *Activity of phrenic motor neurons and diaphragm*: Remains intact during REM sleep.

Cardiovascular system

1. Cardiovascular parameters:
   a. *NREM sleep compared to wake*: ↓ HR, ↓ CO, ↓ BP and =/↓ SVR.
   b. *Tonic REM sleep compared to NREM sleep*: ↓ HR, ↓ CO, ↓ BP and ↓ SVR.

c. *Phasic REM sleep compared to NREM and tonic REM sleep*: ↑ HR, ↑ CO, ↑ BP and ↑ SVR.
d. *During awakenings*: ↑ HR, ↑ CO, ↑ BP and ↑ SVR (due to enhanced sympathetic tone).
2. Nighttime systolic BP is commonly about 10% less than daytime systolic BP ("dipping" phenomenon).
3. Clinical correlation:
   a. Diurnal distribution of ischemic cardiac events and lethal arrhythmias: Peak in the early morning hours (6-11 am).
   b. ↓ Frequency of PVCs during sleep compared to wake. However, ↑ in PVCs during sleep in some persons (e.g., neurological disorders). PVCs are more frequent during REM sleep than NREM sleep.
   c. ↑ Frequency of Prinzmetal angina in the early morning (4-6 am), particularly during REM sleep.

Gastrointestinal system
1. ↓ Swallowing rate.
2. ↓ Salivary production.
3. ↓ Esophageal motility.
4. Circadian rhythmicity in basal gastric acid secretion:
   a. Peak between 10 pm and 2 am.
   b. Nadir between 5 am and 11 am.
5. ↑ Gastric acid secretion during sleep in persons with peptic ulcer disease.
6. ↓ Intestinal motility (i.e., migrating motor complex) and motor tone. ↑ Intestinal motor activity with arousals and awakenings.
7. ↑ Rectal motor activity (with retrograde propagation of contractions that contribute to rectal continence during sleep).
8. ↓ Anal canal pressure.
9. Clinical correlations:
   a. *Gastroesophageal reflux.*
      i. GER is less common during sleep compared to wake.
      ii. Sleep-related GER is associated with more prolonged esophageal acid clearance time and greater duration of mucosal acid contact.
      iii. Prevalence of sleep-related GER is increased in patients with OSA. Optimal PAP therapy may reduce GER symptoms.
   b. *Irritable bowel syndrome.*
      i. Sleep-related conditions: Poor sleep quality in 25-30% of persons (correlated with pain, dyspeptic symptoms and depression).
      ii. PSG features: No significant difference from normal controls.

Renal system
1. ↑ Water reabsorption.
2. ↓ Glomerular filtration.
3. ↑ Renin release (during NREM sleep).
4. Clinical correlations:
   a. ↑ Renal sympathetic nervous system activity and activation of the renin-angiotensin system contribute to BP elevation related to OSA.
   b. Persons with OSA have an increased prevalence of nocturia, which improves with optimal PAP therapy.

Genito-urinary system
1. Penile tumescence (men), and clitoral tumescence and vaginal engorgement (women).

Endocrine system
1. Sleep is enhanced by GHRH, neuropeptide γ and ghrelin.
2. Sleep is inhibited by somatostatin and CRH.

Growth hormone
1. Release of GH occurs primarily during N3 sleep. GH secretion can also occur without N3 sleep (e.g., relaxed supine position). SD may suppress GH secretion.
2. There is one peak in GH secretion (at sleep onset) in men. Several peaks in GH secretion occurring throughout the day and night may be seen in women.
3. GHRH promotes sleep (i.e., ↑ N3 and ↑ R) in men. Somatostatin, by antagonizing GHRH, reduces N3 sleep.
4. Clinical correlations:
   a. ↓ N3 in patients with GH deficiency.
   b. High prevalence of OSA and CSA in acromegaly. Greater likelihood of OSA is related to abnormalities in skeletal structures and soft tissues (e.g., ↑ tongue volume, posterior displacement of the tongue due to vertical facial bone growth, inferior displacement of the hyoid bone, and pharyngeal tissue hypertrophy).
   c. Therapy of acromegaly with surgery (transphenoidal hypophysectomy) or octreotide can improve SRBD.

d. Patients with narcolepsy have higher levels of GH compared to healthy controls.
e. OSA is associated with low levels of GH. GH increases with PAP therapy.
f. With aging, GH decreases due to ↓ N3.

Prolactin
1. Secretion increases during N3 sleep, and decreases during REM sleep. Secretion is suppressed by sleep fragmentation.
2. Secretion is also influenced by circadian rhythms during wakefulness (lower levels at noon and higher levels in the evening).
3. Administration of prolactin increases REM sleep (in animal models).
4. Clinical correlations:
   a. Hyperprolactinoma is associated with ↑ N3.

TSH and thyroid hormone
1. TSH secretion is linked to both sleep and circadian rhythms.
   a. TSH levels are low during the daytime (nadir between 10 am and 7 pm) and increase during the night (between 9 pm and 6 am), with a peak prior to sleep onset.
   b. TSH secretion is inhibited by sleep (particularly N3), and increases with awakenings and SD.
2. ↓ Thyroid hormone levels at night.
3. Clinical correlations:
   a. Insomnia or sleepwalking can develop in persons with hyperthyroidism.
   b. RLS can develop in persons with hypothyroidism.
   c. Hypothyroidism is associated with an increase in apnea index. However, there is no difference in prevalence of hypothyroidism between persons with OSA and healthy individuals. Therefore, routine thyroid function testing in patients with OSA is *not* indicated.
   d. Cardiac ischemia can complicate thyroid therapy for hypothyroidism in persons with untreated OSA.

Parathyroid hormone
1. ↑ Levels during sleep.

CRH, ACTH and cortisol
1. Cortisol secretion is linked primarily to the circadian rhythm rather than to sleep. Cortisol levels begin to rise about 2 hours prior to awakening (peak levels at 8-9 am). Thereafter, cortisol levels decline (nadir at 12 am).
2. Sleep (especially N3) suppresses cortisol secretion.
3. Secretion of cortisol increases during prolonged awakenings (> 20 minutes).
4. CRH inhibits sleep (↓ N3) and enhances vigilance. There is a reciprocal relationship between the effects of GHRH and CRH on sleep.
5. PSG features:
   a. CRH, ACTH or cortisol administration: ↓ R.
   b. CRH administration: ↓ N3.
   c. Cortisol administration: ↑ N3 at low doses. ↑ WASO with higher doses.
6. Clinical correlations:
   a. Cushing disease (↑ levels of cortisol) is associated with ↑ SOL, ↑ WASO and ↓ N3.
   b. Chronic primary insomnia may be associated with higher levels of cortisol and ACTH.
   c. In SWSD, ↑ cortisol levels during daytime sleep, and ↓ cortisol levels during night shift work.
   d. ACTH and cortisol levels increase during SD.

Melatonin
1. Levels rise in the evening, peak in the early morning (between 2-5 am), and decline thereafter, even if no sleep occurs during the night.
2. Synthesis and secretion of melatonin is suppressed by light exposure.

Testosterone
1. Secretion is primarily linked to sleep.
2. ↑ Levels during sleep (young adult men). Peak levels occur about 90 minutes prior to the 1st REM period.
3. Clinical correlations:
   a. ↓ Testosterone levels in patients with OSA. PAP therapy improves testosterone levels.
   b. Polycystic ovarian syndrome is associated with both ↑ testosterone levels and greater risk of OSA.
   c. Administration of testosterone can give rise to ↓ TST and may ↑ AHI (data are conflicting).

Luteinizing hormone
1. ↑ Levels during sleep, mainly during NREM sleep (in adolescents and adult men).
2. LH secretion may remain unchanged or even decline during sleep in adult women, especially during the follicular phase of the menstrual cycle.

Aldosterone
1. ↑ Levels in the early morning prior to awakening.
2. Clinical correlation:
   a. ↑ Aldosterone may be associated with increased risk of OSA.

Antidiuretic hormone
1. ↑ Levels at night.

Renin
1. Secretion is linked to the NREM-REM sleep cycle.
   a. ↑ Levels during NREM sleep (peak levels during N3 sleep).
   b. ↓ Levels during REM sleep.
2. ↑ Levels during recovery sleep following SD.

Atrial natriuretic peptide
1. ↑ Levels in patients with OSA. ↓ Levels with effective PAP therapy.

Insulin
1. ↓ Levels during sleep (insulin secretion may increase during early sleep). Insulin levels are higher in NREM sleep compared to REM sleep. Insulin resistance may develop during SD.
2. OSA increases risk of insulin resistance and type II DM, independent of BMI. Insulin sensitivity improves with PAP therapy.
3. Risk for DM is also increased in patients with narcolepsy.

Leptin
1. Released from peripheral adipocytes. Involved with regulation of energy balance (reduces appetite). *Leptin = lean.*
2. Secretion is influenced by both sleep and circadian rhythms. Greater secretion at night (highest levels from 12 pm to 4 am and lowest levels from 1-2 pm). Secretion declines during sleep restriction.
3. ↑ Levels in persons with OSA (leptin resistance?). Levels decrease with reduction in AHI during PAP therapy.
4. ↓ Levels with loss of nighttime peak in

persons with narcolepsy.

Ghrelin
1. Stimulates appetite and increases food intake. *Ghrelin = gain.*
2. Increases GH secretion.
3. Levels ↑ at night (related to the sleep period) and ↓ during the daytime.
4. Ghrelin promotes N3 sleep.
5. ↑ Levels in some persons with OSA. Levels normalize with optimal PAP therapy.

Neuropeptide γ
1. Neuropeptide γ promotes sleep (↓ SOL and ↑ TST).

Summary of hormone secretion during the night:
1. During the 1st half of the sleep period: ↑ GH, ↓ cortisol and ↓ ACTH.
2. During the 2nd half of the sleep period: ↓ GH, ↑ cortisol and ↑ ACTH.

Musculoskeletal system
1. Sleep is associated with skeletal muscle relaxation (hypotonia or atonia) and inhibition of deep tendon reflexes.
2. Vasoconstriction of skeletal muscle vasculature occurs during REM sleep due to an increase in sympathetic ANS activity.

Pupillary changes
1. Pupillary constriction during NREM and tonic REM sleep, and dilatation during phasic REM sleep.

Immunity
1. Pro-inflammatory cytokines enhance sleep (NREM sleep and delta EEG waves): IL-1β and TNF-α.
   a. Levels of IL-1β and TNF-α increase during sleep.
   b. IL-1β and TNF-α act via nuclear factor-kappa beta [κβ] (NFKB). IL-1β and TNF-α increase, and are increased by, NFKB (positive feedback loop). NFKB, in turn, promotes sleep by enhancing nitric oxide synthase.

IL-1β and TNF-α
⇓⇑
Nuclear factor-κβ
⇓
Nitric oxide synthase

c. Other cytokines that enhance sleep: IL-2, IL-6 and IL-8.
2. Anti-inflammatory cytokines suppress sleep: IL-4, IL-10 and transforming growth factor-beta.
3. Acute infectious and inflammatory processes can give rise to sleepiness.
   a. Response to viral infections: Influenza virus administration results in ↑ NREM and ↓ REM sleep (possibly mediated by IL-1, interferon, GHRH and nitric oxide).
   b. Response to bacterial infections also consists of ↑ NREM and ↓ REM sleep (likely due to lipopolysacccharide [gram – bacteria] or muramyl peptide [gram + bacteria]-induced ↑ in IL-1β, IL-6 and TNF-α). The initial ↑ in NREM sleep may be followed by a subsequent ↓ in NREM sleep.
4. Changes in the immune system in OSA:
   a. ↑ CRP, IL-6 and TNF-α (↓ with PAP therapy). ↓ IL-10.
5. Changes in the immune system in narcolepsy: ↑ IL-6 and ↑ TNF-α.
6. Changes in the immune system in insomnia: Phase advance of peak secretion of IL-6 and TNF-α.

Thermoregulation
1. Neurons in the preoptic and anterior hypothalamus (POAH) are involved with thermoregulation.
   a. Activity of warmth-sensing neurons: ↑ During sleep. ↓ During wake.
   b. Activity of cold-sensing neurons: ↓ During sleep. ↑ During wake.
   c. Mild increases in local POAH temperature: ↓ SOL and ↑ N3 sleep. Activation of POAH warmth-sensing neurons promotes sleep by inhibiting ascending activating systems.
   d. Mild decreases in local POAH temperature: ↑ SOL and ↓ N3 sleep.
2. Core body temperature peaks in the late afternoon and early evening and falls at the onset of sleep. Temperature nadir occurs about 2-4 hours prior to usual wake time.
   a. Peak at 6-8 pm.
   b. Nadir at 4-5 am.
3. Changes in thermoregulation during sleep include:
   a. Fall in core body temperature.
   b. Decline in thermal set point.
   c. Reduced thermoregulatory responses to thermal challenges (↓ During NREM sleep. ↓↓ During REM sleep).
   d. ↓ Metabolic heat production. Loss of heat production from shivering during REM sleep.
   e. ↑ Heat loss (due to sweating and peripheral vasodilatation).
4. Sleep latency and architecture are influenced by changes in body temperature at bedtime.
   a. Exposure to extreme hot or cold environmental temperatures suppresses sleep onset and causes sleep disruption.
      i. In contrast, mild whole-body warming 1-2 hours before bedtime can enhance sleep (due to mild activation of heat response mechanisms).
   b. Nocturnal sleep typically occurs during the falling phase of the temperature rhythm (after CTmax).
   c. Awakening occurs during the rising phase of the temperature rhythm (after CTmin).
   d. Initiating sleep during the falling phase of the temperature rhythm: ↓ SOL, ↑ TST and ↑ N3.
      i. High distal-to-proximal skin temperature gradient (i.e., warmer extremities and cooler body suggestive of greater heat loss response) is associated with ↓ SOL, ↓ WASO and ↑ N3 sleep.
   e. Initiating sleep during the rising phase of the temperature rhythm: ↑ SOL, ↓ TST, ↓ N3 and ↑ R.
   f. Useful reminder:
      Cool down to sleep sound.
      Heat up to wake up.
5. Clinical correlations:
   a. Insomnia (sleep-onset): Phase delay of body temperature rhythm with attempts to sleep occurring nearer to CTmax.
   b. Mood disorder: Reduced temperature rhythm amplitude and decreased body temperature at bedtime.

Metabolism
1. Metabolic rate decreases during NREM sleep compared to wake.
2. Metabolic rate during REM sleep is either similar to or greater than during NREM sleep.
3. Thus, a useful reminder: *Wake > NREM ≤ REM.*

Dreaming

1. Dreams can occur during both REM (accounting for 80% of dreams) and NREM (20% of dreams) sleep.
2. Compared to REM sleep-related dreams that tend to be more complex and irrational, NREM dreams are generally simpler and more realistic.

Summary: what goes up and what goes down during sleep

1. *What goes up during sleep:*
   a. *Parasympathetic activity.*
   b. *$PaCO_2$.*
   c. *Renal water reabsorption.*
   d. *Hormone secretion:*
      i. *Growth hormone (during N3 sleep).*
      ii. *Prolactin (during N3 sleep).*
      iii. *Parathyroid hormone.*
      iv. *Renin (during NREM sleep).*
      v. *Antidiuretic hormone.*
      vi. *Testosterone.*
2. *What goes down during sleep:*
   a. *Sympathetic activity.*
   b. *PaO_2 and SaO_2.*
   c. *Tidal volume and minute ventilation.*
   d. *Hypoxic and hypercapnic ventilatory responses.*
   e. *UA dilator muscle tone.*
   f. *Activity of accessory muscles of respiration.*
   g. *HR, CO and BP (NREM and tonic REM sleep).*
   h. *Frequency of PVCs.*
   i. *Swallowing rate and salivary production.*
   j. *Esophageal and intestinal motility.*
   k. *Glomerular filtration.*
   l. *Hormonal secretion:*
      i. *Cortisol (levels decrease during N3 sleep).*
      ii. *Insulin.*
   m. *Muscle tone.*
   n. *Core body temperature and thermoregulatory responses to thermal challenges.*
   o. *Metabolic rate (during NREM sleep).*

Sleep Deprivation: Consequences

In this section
Key concepts
General
Central nervous system
Autonomic nervous system
Cognition
Respiratory system
Cardiovascular system
Endocrine system
Metabolism
Immune system
Ocular changes
Behavioral and psychiatric effects
Miscellaneous effects
PSG features
Waking EEG features
Animal models
Summary: what goes up and what goes down during sleep deprivation

Key concepts
1. Vulnerability to SD varies within individuals across time (state instability) and between individuals (differential tolerance).
2. The physiological and neurocognitive consequences of total SD appear to differ in some ways from those of chronic sleep restriction.
3. Persons often underestimate the negative impact of SD on cognition and performance.
4. Older adults are more resilient to SD compared to younger adults.

General
1. ↑ Morbidity.
2. ↑ Mortality (with TST either < 6.5 or > 7.5 hours per night): Mechanism unknown.
3. ↑ Sleepiness.
4. ↓ Vigilance.
5. ↓ Vigor.
6. Hypothermia (severe SD).

Central nervous system
1. ↓ Pain tolerance.
2. ↓ Seizure threshold.
3. Hyperactive gag and deep tendon reflexes.
4. Nystagmus.
5. Ptosis.
6. Sluggish corneal reflexes.
7. Slurring of speech.
8. Tremors.
9. ↓ Cerebral glucose metabolism (particularly subcortical frontal and mid-brain regions).

Autonomic nervous system
1. ↑ Sympathetic activity.

Cognition
1. ↓ Cognitive performance.
2. ↓ Attention.
3. Impairment of working memory and executive function.
4. Impairment of information-processing and decision-making.
5. Slowing of response time.
6. Hyperactivity in children.

Respiratory system
1. ↓ FEV_1 and FVC.
2. ↓ Ventilatory responsiveness.

Cardiovascular system
1. ↑ Risk of coronary events (if TST is < 6 hours).

Endocrine system
1. ↑ Cortisol and ACTH (evening levels).
2. ↓ GH.
3. ↑ Ghrelin.
4. ↑ Insulin resistance (↓ glucose tolerance).
5. ↓ Leptin activity.
6. ↓ Prolactin.
7. ↓ Thyroid hormone.

*Useful reminder: **LL-GG** (lower leptin, greater ghrelin) seen in SD.*

Metabolism
1. ↑ Hunger and appetite (preference for salty, sweet and starchy foods).
2. ↑ Caloric intake.
3. Weight gain (weight loss in late stages of profound SD).
4. ↑ Risk of obesity.
5. ↑ Metabolic rate.

Immune system
1. ↑ IL-1, IL-6, CRP and TNF-α.
2. ↓ Antibody titers to influenza and hepatitis A vaccination acutely.
3. ↓ Febrile response to endotoxin.
4. ↓ Resistance to infection (presence of bacteria in sterile areas of body). Animal research: ↑ Translocation of bacteria across the gut wall.
5. Reduction in CD4, CD16, CD56 and CD57 lymphocytes.

Ocular changes
1. ↓ Saccadic velocity.
2. ↑ Slow eye movements.
3. ↑ Slow eyelid closures.

Behavioral and psychiatric effects
1. Negative impact on mood.
2. Remission of major depressive disorder (in ≈ 50% of patients).

Miscellaneous effects
1. ↑ Medical errors (omission and commission).
2. ↑ Motor vehicle accidents (↑ Rate of accidents on a driving simulator).

PSG features
1. ↓ SOL (also seen in the MSLT).
2. ↑ TST.
3. ↑ Slow wave EEG activity.
4. ↑ N3 (1st night after SD).
5. ↓ Sleep spindles.
6. ↓ REM SL.
7. ↑ R (2nd night after SD).
Note: Sleep architecture generally normalizes by the 3rd night of recovery sleep.

Waking EEG features
1. Shift to slower EEG frequencies (i.e., theta [4-7 Hz] and delta [< 4 Hz] waves).

Animal models
1. ↑ Homeostatic sleep drive.
2. Failure of thermoregulation.
3. ↓ Response to infectious agents.
4. ↑ Metabolic rate.
5. Weight loss despite increased food intake.
6. ↑ Norepinephrine level.
7. Skin lesions.
8. Death during prolonged SD.

Summary: what goes up and what goes down during sleep deprivation
1. *What goes up during SD:*
   a. *Sleepiness.*
   b. *Sympathetic activity.*
   c. *Hormones:*
      i. *Cortisol and ACTH.*
      ii. *Ghrelin.*
      iii. *Norepinephrine.*
   d. *Insulin resistance.*
   e. *Metabolic rate.*
   f. *Medical errors and motor vehicle accidents.*

2. *What goes down during SD:*
   a. *Vigilance.*
   b. *Pain tolerance.*
   c. *Seizure threshold.*
   d. *Cognition and attention.*
   e. *Hormones:*
      i. *Growth hormone.*
      ii. *Leptin activity.*
      iii. *Prolactin.*
      iv. *Thyroid hormone.*
   f. *Antibody titers to influenza and hepatitis A vaccination acutely.*
   g. *Febrile response to endotoxin.*
   h. *Resistance to infection.*

Sleep-Wake Regulation

General

1. Biological rhythms are ubiquitous and are characterized by specific frequency (number of oscillations per unit time), period length (interval between 2 consecutive events), amplitude (maximal excursion from peak to trough) and phase (temporal position in relation to an external cue).
2. A *circadian* rhythm consists of 1 oscillation approximately every 24 hours.
3. Circadian rhythms free-run at a genetically determined frequency, which is generally slightly over 24 hours (most commonly about 24.2 hours). This endogenous circadian period is referred to as "*tau*".
4. Entrainment adjusts and synchronizes the endogenous circadian rhythm to the external 24-hour period, using environmental cues called *zeitgebers*. These external stimuli can either be photic (dominant synchronizer) or nonphotic (e.g., meals or activity). *Phase advance* refers to a shift of the circadian period to an earlier time in the 24-hour cycle, whereas *phase delay* involves a shift of the period to a later time in the 24-hour cycle.

Control of sleep and waking

1. Two basic intrinsic components interact to regulate the timing and consolidation of sleep and wake:
   a. Sleep homeostasis: Dependent on the sleep-wake cycle.
   b. Circadian rhythm: Independent of the sleep-wake cycle.
2. These two processes influence sleep latency, duration and quality.
3. Timing of sleep is also determined by behavioral influences (e.g., social activities and work schedules).

Biological rhythm markers

1. Two biological markers are used to estimate the timing of circadian rhythms, namely DLMO and CTmin.
2. DLMO is the time when melatonin levels start to rise, normally occurring 2-3 hours before bedtime.
3. CTmin usually occurs 2-4 hours before the end of the sleep period.

Sleep homeostasis

1. An increase in sleep pressure that is related to the duration of prior wakefulness (i.e., the longer a person is awake, the sleepier one becomes).
2. Sleep pressure declines following a sufficient duration of sleep time.
3. Adenosine, a neurotransmitter, likely has a major role in sleep homeostasis.

Circadian neurosystem

1. Its main role is to promote wakefulness during the day.
2. There are 2 circadian rhythm-related peaks in wakefulness (wake-maintenance zones): Late morning and early evening.
3. There are 2 periods of circadian troughs in alertness (increased sleep propensity): Early morning and early-mid afternoon.

Control of circadian rhythms

1. Circadian rhythms are controlled by transcription-translation positive and negative feedback loops involving positive, negative and regulatory components.
   a. Positive components: *Clock* and *Bmal1*.
   b. Negative components: *Period, Cryptochrome* and *Timeless*.

c. Regulatory components: *Casein kinase 1 epsilon*.
2. Circadian gene feedback loops: Transcription of *Clock* and *Bmal1* genes into mRNA ⇒ Translation of *Clock* and *Bmal1* mRNA into proteins ⇒ Translocation of Clock and Bmal1 proteins into the nucleus ⇒ Activation of transcription and translation of *Period*, *Cryptochrome* and *Timeless* that are then translocated into the nucleus ⇒ Inhibition of Clock and Bmal1.

Circadian timing systems
1. The SCN in the anterior hypothalamus (above the optic chiasm) is the master circadian rhythm generator in mammals.
2. It is likely that other anatomical sites may also harbor endogenous clocks.

Suprachiasmatic nuclei
1. Activity is independent of the environment, firing more frequently during the daytime than at night.
2. Actions of the SCN include: (a) promotion of wakefulness during the day, and (b) consolidation of sleep during the night.
3. Ablation of the SCN results in random distribution of sleep throughout the day and night as well as reduction in duration of waking periods (in some).

Regions of the SCN
1. The SCN consists of two regions, namely a core and a shell region.
2. Core region:
   a. Location: Ventrolateral.
   b. Neurotransmitter: Vasoactive intestinal peptide.
   c. Size of neurons: Small ($30~\mu m^2$).
   d. Function: Resets endogenous circadian rhythms.
3. Shell region:
   a. Location: Dorsomedial.
   b. Neurotransmitter: Arginine vasopressin.
   c. Size of neurons: Large ($45~\mu m^2$).
   d. Function: Maintains endogenous circadian rhythms.

Afferent SCN pathways
1. There are several afferent inputs, both photic and non-photic, to the SCN.
2. Glutamatergic:
   a. Photic stimuli.
   b. Main afferent connection.
   c. Eyes (photosensitive retina ganglion cells containing the photopigment, melanopsin) ⇒ retinohypothalamic tract ⇒ SCN.
   d. Neurotransmitters: Glutamate and pituitary adenylate cyclase-activating polypeptide.
   e. Retinal photoreceptors are most sensitive to shorter wavelength light (from 450 nm [blue] to 500 nm [blue-green]).
3. Alternate afferent connection:
   a. Photic stimuli.
   b. Thalamic intergeniculate leaflet of the lateral geniculate nuclei ⇒ geniculohypothalamic tract ⇒ SCN.
   c. Neurotransmitters: Neuropeptide γ and GABA.
   d. Light entrainment is lost with disruption of the retinohypothalamic tract but not with interruption of the alternate geniculohypothalamic tract.
4. Histaminergic:
   a. Photic stimuli.
   b. From the tuberomammillary neurons in the posterior hypothalamus.
   c. Neurotransmitter: Histamine.
5. Cholinergic:
   a. Photic stimuli.
   b. From the basal forebrain and brainstem.
   c. Neurotransmitter: Acetylcholine.
6. Serotonergic:
   a. Non-photic stimuli.
   b. From the midbrain median raphe nuclei.
   c. Neurotransmitter: Serotonin.

Efferent SCN projections
1. The SCN has efferent projections to the basal forebrain, hypocretin neurons, hypothalamus, locus ceruleus, pineal gland, thalamus and ventrolateral preoptic nucleus.
2. Neurotransmitters: Transforming growth factor-α and prokineticin 2.
3. Neural pathway from the SCN to the pineal gland: SCN ⇒ hypothalamus (para/subventricular nuclei) ⇒ medial forebrain bundle ⇒ spinal cord (intermediolateral gray column neurons) ⇒ superior cervical ganglion ⇒ pineal gland.

Melatonin
1. Synthesized and released by the pineal gland: Tryptophan ⇒ serotonin (5-hydroxytryptamine) ⇒ melatonin (N-acetyl-5-methoxytryptamine).

2. Greatest secretion at night. Secretion is inhibited by light exposure.
3. Influence of melatonin on the SCN:
   a. Phase delay circadian sleep-wake rhythm when taken in the morning.
   b. Phase advance circadian sleep-wake rhythm when given in the afternoon or early evening.
   c. Less effective in phase shifting circadian rhythms than light exposure.
4. There are 2 melatonin receptors:
   a. MT1: Acts to inhibit firing of SCN.
   b. MT2: Phase-shifting action.
5. Also possess mild hypnotic properties.

Differential Diagnoses

In this section
Excessive sleepiness
Transient insomnia
Chronic insomnia
Sleep-onset insomnia
Sleep-onset insomnia in children
Sleep-maintenance insomnia
Sleep-maintenance insomnia in children
Early morning awakenings
Persistently short nocturnal sleep duration
Vivid and disturbed dreaming
Unusual behavior or activity during sleep
Nighttime automatic behavior
Sleep paralysis
Nocturnal limb movements
Body movements at sleep onset
Sound production
Vocalizations during sleep
Oral movements
Nighttime sensation of obstruction in upper airway or GI tract
Dyspnea or choking during sleep
Nighttime eating
Cataplexy-like features
Nocturnal oxygen desaturation

Excessive sleepiness
1. Circadian rhythm sleep disorders.
   a. Advanced sleep phase disorder.
   b. Delayed sleep phase disorder.
   c. Free running disorder.
   d. Irregular sleep wake rhythm.
   e. Jet lag.
   f. Shift work sleep disorder.
2. Idiopathic hypersomnia.
3. Insufficient sleep syndrome.
4. Long sleeper (when following conventional sleep duration).
5. Medical, neurological and psychiatric disorders.
   a. Chronic renal failure.
   b. Hepatic encephalopathy.
   c. Sleeping sickness.
   d. Prader-Willi syndrome.
   e. Brain tumors.
   f. Dementia.
   g. Hydrocephalus.
   h. Parkinson disease.
   i. Encephalitis.
   j. Stroke.
   k. Mood disorder.
6. Medication or substance use or withdrawal.
7. Narcolepsy.
8. Obstructive and central sleep apnea.
9. Periodic limb movement disorder.
10. Post-traumatic hypersomnia (head injury).
11. Recurrent hypersomnia.
    a. Kleine-Levin syndrome.
    b. Menstrual-associated hypersomnia.

Transient insomnia
1. Acute stressors.
2. Jet lag.
3. Medication and substance use.
4. Shift work.

Chronic insomnia
1. *Primary:*
   a. Idiopathic insomnia.
   b. Paradoxical insomnia.
   c. Psychophysiologic insomnia.
2. *Secondary:*
   a. Behavioral disorders.
      i. Inadequate sleep hygiene.
      ii. Limit-setting sleep disorder.
      iii. Sleep-onset association disorder.
   b. Circadian rhythm sleep disorders.
      i. Advanced sleep phase disorder.
      ii. Delayed sleep phase disorder.
      iii. Free running rhythm.
      iv. Irregular sleep wake rhythm.
      v. Shift work sleep disorder.

c. Environmental factors.
   i. Altitude insomnia.
   ii. Environmental sleep disorder.
   iii. Food allergy insomnia.
   iv. Toxin-induced sleep disorder.
d. Primary sleep disorders.
   i. Central sleep apnea.
   ii. Obstructive sleep apnea.
   iii. Nocturnal leg cramps.
   iv. Nightmares.
   v. Periodic limb movement disorder.
   vi. Restless legs syndrome.
e. Medical disorders.
   i. Cancer.
   ii. Cardiac disorders (nocturnal angina or CHF).
   iii. Dermatologic disorders (pruritus).
   iv. Gastrointestinal disorders.
   v. Infectious disorders (AIDS).
   vi. Nocturia.
   vii. Pain syndromes, chronic.
   viii. Renal failure.
   ix. Respiratory disorders (asthma, COPD or CCAHS).
f. Neurological disorders.
   i. Cerebral degenerative disorders.
   ii. Dementia.
   iii. Fatal familial insomnia.
   iv. Nocturnal paroxysmal dystonia.
   v. Parkinson disease.
   vi. Sleep-related headaches.
   vii. Sleep-related seizures.
g. Psychiatric disorders.
   i. Alcoholism.
   ii. Anxiety disorders.
   iii. Mood disorders.
   iv. Panic disorders.
   v. Personality disorders.
   vi. Post-traumatic stress disorder.
   vii. Schizophrenia.
   viii. Somatoform disorders.
h. Menstruation, pregnancy and menopause.
i. Medication or substance use.

Sleep-onset insomnia
1. Adjustment sleep disorder.
2. Altitude insomnia.
3. Circadian rhythm sleep disorders.
   a. Delayed sleep phase disorder.
   b. Free running disorder.
   c. Irregular sleep wake rhythm.
   d. Shift work sleep disorder.
4. Environmental sleep disorder.
5. Idiopathic insomnia.
6. Inadequate sleep hygiene.

7. Paradoxical insomnia.
8. Psychiatric disorders.
   a. Anxiety disorders.
   b. Mood disorders.
   c. Post-traumatic stress disorder.
9. Psychophysiologic insomnia.
10. Restless legs syndrome.
11. Substance use or withdrawal (stimulants).

Sleep-onset insomnia in children
1. Adjustment sleep disorder.
2. Bedtime resistance.
3. Behavioral and psychiatric disorders.
   a. Anxiety disorders.
   b. Attention deficit-hyperactivity disorder.
   c. Mood disorders.
   d. Post-traumatic stress disorder.
4. Colic.
5. Delayed sleep phase disorder.
6. Environmental sleep disorder.
7. Food allergy insomnia.
8. Inadequate sleep hygiene.
9. Limit-setting sleep disorder.
10. Medical disorders.
11. Nighttime fears (fear of darkness or being left alone).
12. Psychophysiologic insomnia.
13. Restless legs syndrome.
14. Separation anxiety.
15. Sleep-onset association disorder.
16. Variable sleep schedule.

Sleep-maintenance insomnia
1. Alcohol (withdrawal from).
2. Medical, neurological and psychiatric disorders.
   a. Chronic obstructive pulmonary disease.
   b. Congestive heart failure.
   c. Gastroesophageal reflux disease.
   d. Mood and panic disorders.
   e. Nocturnal asthma.
3. Primary sleep disorders.
   a. Central sleep apnea.
   b. Obstructive sleep apnea.
   c. Parasomnias.
   d. Periodic limb movement disorder.
   e. Psychophysiologic insomnia.

Sleep-maintenance insomnia in children
1. Colic.
2. Inadequate sleep hygiene.
3. Medical disorders.
4. Obstructive sleep apnea.
5. Parasomnias (nightmares).
6. Periodic limb movement disorder.
7. Psychophysiologic insomnia.

Early morning awakenings
1. Alcohol (withdrawal from).
2. Advanced sleep phase disorder.
3. Depression.
4. Withdrawal from short-acting hypnotic agents.

Persistently short nocturnal sleep duration
1. Fatal familial insomnia.
2. Idiopathic insomnia.
3. Inadequate sleep hygiene.
4. Manic phase of bipolar disorder.
5. Polyphasic sleep with frequent daytime napping.
6. Psychophysiologic insomnia.
7. Short sleeper.
8. Stimulant use or abuse.

Vivid and disturbed dreaming
1. Alcohol (withdrawal from).
2. Isolated sleep paralysis.
3. Medication and substance use (e.g., beta blockers).
4. Nightmares.
5. Nocturnal panic attacks.
6. Obstructive sleep apnea.
7. Post-traumatic stress disorder.
8. REM sleep behavior disorder.
9. Schizophrenia.
10. Terrifying hypnagogic hallucinations.

Unusual behavior or activity during sleep
1. Malingering.
2. Medication, substance or alcohol use.
3. Nocturnal paroxysmal dystonia.
4. Nocturnal psychogenic dissociative disorders.
5. Nocturnal seizures.
6. Obstructive sleep apnea.
7. Panic attacks.
8. Parasomnias.
   a. Nightmares.
   b. REM sleep behavior disorder.
   c. Rhythmic movement disorders.
   d. Sleep terrors.
   e. Sleepwalking.
9. Periodic limb movement disorder.
10. Post-traumatic stress disorder.

Nighttime automatic behavior
1. Dissociative and fugue-like states.
2. Malingering.
3. Medication, substance or alcohol use.
4. Narcolepsy.
5. Obstructive sleep apnea.
6. Parasomnias.

7. Seizures (especially partial complex).
8. Sleep deprivation.

Sleep paralysis
1. Catatonia.
2. Familial (X-linked dominant) sleep paralysis.
3. Isolated sleep paralysis.
4. Narcolepsy.
5. Seizures (atonic).
6. Sleep deprivation.
7. Transient (hyperkalemic or hypokalemic) paralysis.

Nocturnal limb movements
1. Fragmentary myoclonus.
2. Neurodegenerative disorders (e.g., PD).
3. Nocturnal seizures.
4. Obstructive sleep apnea-related arousals.
5. Periodic limb movements of sleep.
6. Phasic movements during REM sleep.
7. REM sleep behavior disorder.
8. Rhythmic movement disorder.
9. Sleep starts.

Body movements at sleep onset
1. Periodic limb movements of sleep.
2. Propriospinal myoclonus.
3. Restless legs syndrome.
4. Rhythmic movement sleep disorder.
5. Sleep starts.

Sound production
1. Bruxism.
2. Catathrenia.
3. Confusional arousal.
4. Nightmare.
5. Obstructive sleep apnea-related grunting.
6. REM sleep behavior disorder.
7. Seizures.
8. Sleep talking.
9. Sleep terrors.
10. Snoring.
11. Stridor (due to UA narrowing).
12. Wheezing.

Vocalizations during sleep
1. Confusional arousal.
2. Nightmares.
3. Nocturnal seizures.
4. REM sleep behavior disorder.
5. Sleep talking.
6. Sleep terror.

Oral movements
1. Facial mandibular myoclonus.
2. Rhythmic movement disorder.

3. Seizures.
4. Sleep bruxism.

Nighttime sensation of obstruction in upper airway or GI tract
1. Gastroesophageal reflux (+/- aspiration).
2. Obstructive sleep apnea.
3. Panic disorder.
4. Sleep-related choking syndrome.
5. Sleep-related abnormal swallowing syndrome.
6. Sleep-related laryngospasm.
7. Sleep terrors.

Dyspnea or choking during sleep
1. Chronic obstructive pulmonary disease.
2. Gastroesophageal reflux (+/- aspiration).
3. Heart failure (paroxysmal nocturnal dyspnea).
4. Nocturnal asthma.
5. Obstructive sleep apnea.
6. Panic disorder.
7. Sleep-related choking syndrome.
8. Sleep-related laryngospasm.
9. Sudden unexplained nocturnal death syndrome.

Nighttime eating
1. Hypoglycemia.
2. Kleine-Levin syndrome (recurrent EDS, hypersexuality and hyperphagia).

3. Medication induced (e.g., zolpidem and related drugs).
4. Obstructive sleep apnea.
5. Peptic ulcer disease.
6. Sleep-related eating disorder.

Cataplexy-like features
1. Arrhythmias.
2. Conversion disorder.
3. Malingering.
4. Neuromuscular weakness.
5. Orthostatic hypotension.
6. Periodic paralysis.
7. Psychosis.
8. Seizure (partial complex, atonic or absence).
9. Syncope.
10. Transient ischemic attack.
11. Vestibular dysfunction.

Nocturnal oxygen desaturation
1. Altitude (high).
2. Alveolar hypoventilation syndromes.
3. Central sleep apnea.
4. Chronic obstructive pulmonary disease.
5. Congestive heart failure.
6. Diaphragm paralysis.
7. Neuromuscular disorders.
8. Nocturnal asthma.
9. Obstructive sleep apnea.
10. Restrictive lung disease.

Sleepless Nights

General

1. Insomnia is a disorder characterized by repeated difficulty with either falling or staying asleep, despite adequate opportunity, condition and time to do so. Associated with impairment of daytime function and occurs ≥ 3 nights a week.
    a. *Sleep-onset insomnia* - Difficulty falling asleep.

b. *Sleep-maintenance insomnia* - Frequent or prolonged awakenings.
c. *Terminal insomnia* - Final morning awakening that is earlier than desired.
d. *Nonrestorative sleep* - Unrefreshed feeling upon awakening.
2. Persons with insomnia often report greater subjective estimates of sleep disturbance compared to objective PSG measures of sleep. They may overestimate SOL and underestimate TST.
3. General changes in sleep architecture: (1) SOL $\geq$ 30 minutes, (2) WASO $\geq$ 30 minutes, (3) SE < 85%, or (4) TST < 6-6.5 hours.
4. Many persons with insomnia have either an underlying psychiatric pathology, or an increased risk of developing a new-onset psychiatric illness.

Demographics
1. Insomnia is the most common sleep disorder.
2. About 30-50% of adults report occasional insomnia. An estimated 10-30% of adults complain of chronic insomnia.
3. Prevalence is greater among older adults, shift workers, and persons who are poor, widowed or divorced.
4. Gender: F > M.

Pathophysiologic model of insomnia
1. Factors related to the development and maintenance of sleep disturbance can be classified into three groups (Spielman's model).
   a. *Predisposing factors* that increase the likelihood of developing insomnia (e.g., physiologic or psychological hyperarousal; or decreased homeostatic sleep drive). These factors are present prior to the start of insomnia.
   b. *Precipitating factors* that trigger the start of insomnia (e.g., changes in sleep environment or sleep-wake schedule; acute illness; or stressful life events).
   c. *Perpetuating factors* that sustain the sleep disturbance (even after the initial precipitating factor has resolved). These include substance or medication use, poor sleep hygiene, or maladaptive behaviors related to sleep.

Pathophysiology of sleep disturbance
1. There are several mechanisms that are responsible for sleep disturbance in persons with insomnia. These include:
   a. Somatic and cognitive hyperarousal.
      i. Greater sympathetic ANS tone.
      ii. Higher metabolic rates (including cerebral hypermetabolism, $\uparrow$ HR and $\uparrow$ body temperature).
   b. Persistent sensory perception and information processing.
   c. Intrinsic sleep instability.
      i. Cyclic alternating EEG patterns.
      ii. Greater high-frequency EEG activity during sleep.
   d. Later CTmin (compared to good sleepers).
   e. Circadian dysrhythmia.
   f. Dysregulation of homeostatic sleep drive.
   g. Dysfunctional cognitive processes: Prone to worry, unreasonable expectations about need for sleep, and unrealistic concerns about consequences of lack of sleep.

Risk factors for insomnia
1. Female gender.
2. Advancing age.
3. Lower socioeconomic status or unemployment.
4. Marital status (divorced or widowed).
5. Shift work.
6. Poor health status and physical disability.
7. Medical, neurological and psychiatric disorders (e.g., respiratory disorders, dementia, anxiety, depression and schizophrenia).

Consequences of insomnia
1. $\uparrow$ Likelihood of accidents.
2. $\uparrow$ Risk of developing a psychiatric illness (e.g., depression).
3. $\uparrow$ Subjective sleepiness (especially during acute insomnia). Objective measures (i.e., MSLT) generally do not demonstrate significant EDS.
4. Fatigue.
5. Cognitive impairment (memory, attention and concentration).
6. Impaired academic and occupational performance.
7. $\uparrow$ Absenteeism.
8. Chronic hypnotic use (especially in women and older adults).
9. $\downarrow$ QOL.
10. $\uparrow$ Healthcare utilization.

Classification of insomnia based on duration of sleep disturbance

1. *Transient insomnia*: Lasting only a few days.
2. *Chronic insomnia*: Persisting for more than 1-3 months.

Classification of insomnia based on etiology of sleep disturbance

1. *Primary (idiopathic) insomnia*: Not related to any underlying medical, neurological or psychiatric disorder, or medication use, abuse or withdrawal.
   a. Includes Idiopathic insomnia, Paradoxical insomnia and Psychophysiologic insomnia.
2. *Comorbid insomnia*: Associated with a medical, neurological or psychiatric disorder, or medication use, abuse or withdrawal.

Common causes of chronic insomnia

1. Psychiatric disorders: 35-40% of cases of insomnia.
2. Psychophysiologic insomnia: 15%.
3. Alcohol and drug use: 3-12%.
4. RLS: 8-12%.
5. OSA: 5-6%.

Specific causes of insomnia

1. Adjustment insomnia.
2. Altitude insomnia.
3. Behavioral insomnia of childhood.
   a. Limit-setting sleep disorder.
   b. Sleep-onset association insomnia.
4. Familial fatal insomnia.
5. Food allergy insomnia.
6. Idiopathic insomnia.
7. Inadequate sleep hygiene.
8. Paradoxical insomnia (sleep state misperception).
9. Psychophysiologic insomnia.

Adjustment insomnia

1. Sleep disturbance due to an identifiable acute stressor (e.g., momentous life event, change in sleeping environment, or an acute illness). Duration of insomnia is < 3 months. Sleep normalizes with resolution of the acute stressor or once the individual adapts sufficiently to the stressor.
2. Gender: F > M. Prevalence greater among older adults.
3. Useful factoid:
   a. Another disorder (e.g., psychophysiologic insomnia) should be considered if insomnia persists beyond 3 months.

Altitude insomnia

1. Sleep disturbance develops during ascent (> 2000-4000 meters) due to periodic breathing during sleep as a result of hypoxia and respiratory alkalosis. Arousals can occur during the hyperpneic phase of periodic breathing.
2. Symptoms resolve with acclimatization or after descent to lower altitudes.
3. Therapy:
   a. O_2 therapy may decrease periodic breathing but does not consistently improve sleep quality.
   b. Acetazolamide stimulates respiration via production of metabolic acidosis. It improves hypoxemia, periodic breathing and sleep quality.

Behavioral insomnia of childhood

1. Can be either *limit-setting type* (bedtime resistance due to inadequate enforcement of bedtime by caregiver), or *sleep-onset association type* (problematic associations required for sleep to occur).
2. Diagnosed in children > 6 months of age. Prevalence in children: 10-30%. Gender: M > F (uncertain).
3. Limit-setting sleep disorder:
   a. Repetitive stalling or refusal to go to sleep at an *appropriate* time when requested to do so.
   b. Sleep comes naturally and quickly when limits to further activities are strictly enforced.
   c. Seen in children ≥ 2 years of age who start to develop verbal communication skills.
   d. PSG: Normal sleep architecture.
4. Sleep-onset association disorder:
   a. Inability to fall asleep unless certain desired conditions (e.g., favorite toy or presence of a caregiver) are present at bedtime.
   b. May persist into adulthood.
   c. PSG features:
      i. When required associations are absent: ↑ SOL and ↑ WASO.
      ii. When required associations are present: Normal sleep architecture.

Fatal familial insomnia

1. Autosomal dominant disorder secondary to a prion disease.
2. Progressive sleep disturbance and insomnia, with sleep loss eventually

becoming total. Terminates in stupor, coma and death generally within 12 months to a few years after its onset.
   a. Vivid dreaming and spontaneous lapses into a dreamlike state (oneiric stupor) with motor activity.
3. The hereditary form is due to a GAC to AAC mutation (substitution of aspartic acid with asparagine) at codon 178 of the prion PRNP gene at chromosome 20. This cosegregates with a methionine polymorphism at codon 129.
   a. Useful n4mation:
      i. Interestingly, the familial form of Creutzfeldt-Jakob disease, another prion disease, results from a similar mutation at codon 178 but with coding for valine by codon 129 on the mutated allele.
      ii. Cases of sporadic fatal insomnia do not demonstrate the mutation at codon 178 but possess the codon 129-methionine polymorphism on both alleles.
4. Classification of FFI based on methionine polymorphism at codon 129:
   a. Methionine homozygous:
      i. Disease course: Short.
      ii. Duration of survival: < 12 months.
   b. Methionine-valine heterozygous:
      i. Disease course: Longer.
      ii. Duration of survival: 1-6 years.
5. Associated features:
   a. Loss of circadian rhythms of body temperature, hemodynamic parameters and endocrine hormones.
   b. Autonomic hyperactivity (hyperthermia, hypertension, excessive salivation and sweating).
   c. Neurological abnormalities (myoclonus, tremors, hallucinations, dystonia, ataxia and dysarthria).
   d. Tachypnea and dyspnea.
   e. Generalized body wasting (in terminal stage).
6. Rare condition. Onset during adulthood. Gender: M = F.
7. Pathologic features:
   a. Degeneration and reactive gliosis of thalamic nuclei (anterior ventral and dorsomedial) and inferior olivary nucleus. No associated inflammation. Thalamic hypometabolism on PET scanning.
   b. Grey matter deposition of proteinase K-resistant prion protein type 2.

8. Complications:
   a. Infections: Respiratory and urinary tract.
   b. Dysphagia.
9. PSG features:
   a. In early stages, periods of wakefulness alternate with EEG desynchronization, bursts of REM activity and loss of muscle tone.
   b. Progressive loss of sleep spindles, K complexes and delta waves. Fragmentation of REM sleep, which may occur without muscle atonia.
   c. Flattening and unreactive EEG in terminal disease.
10. No known specific therapy.

Food allergy insomnia
1. Sleep disturbance develops as a result of ingestion of a specific food or drink. Other symptoms of allergy (e.g., rash or gastrointestinal discomfort) may also be present.

Idiopathic insomnia
1. Longstanding insomnia that is not associated with any identifiable etiology.
2. Prevalence of 0.7% in adolescents and 1% in young adults. Accounts for < 10% of persons with complaints of insomnia presenting to the sleep clinics.
3. Onset during infancy or early childhood. Chronic life-long course without periods of remission. Increased risk of developing major depression.
4. Diagnosis by clinical history (i.e., exclusion of other causes of sleep disturbance) and sleep diaries. PSG is not routinely indicated.

Inadequate sleep hygiene
1. Sleep disturbance due to activities or behavior that increase arousal or decrease sleep propensity, and that are under a person's control.

Paradoxical insomnia (sleep state misperception)
1. Subjective reports of chronic severe insomnia (very minimal or no sleep) during most nights associated with no PSG evidence of significant sleep disturbance. Patients often overestimate SOL and underestimate TST compared to objective measures of sleep.
2. No daytime napping or impairment of daytime functioning.
3. Accounts for < 5% of cases of chronic

insomnia.
4. Onset commonly during early to mid-adulthood. Gender: F > M.
5. Chronic course.
6. PSG features: Normal or near normal SOL, sleep quality and sleep architecture despite subjective reports of minimal or no sleep during PSG.
    a. Often, TST > 6.5 hours.
    b. MSLT: Normal or suggests mild sleepiness.

Psychophysiologic insomnia
1. Chronic (≥ 1 month) sleep disturbance secondary to heightened cognitive (rumination and intrusive thoughts) and somatic (increased agitation and muscle tone) arousal at bedtime. Learned maladaptive sleep-preventing behavior. Excessive anxiety and frustration about inability to sleep. Conditioned arousal is limited to a person's own bed and bedroom (sleep is frequently better in another room).
2. Prevalence of 1-2% in the general population. Accounts for 15% of cases of chronic insomnia. Onset generally during adolescence or early adulthood. Gender: F > M.
3. Chronic course that may progressively worsen if untreated. Increased risk of developing depression.
4. Diagnosis by clinical history. PSG is not routinely indicated. "First-night effect" and "reverse first-night effect" (worse or better sleep than usual during the first sleep laboratory night, respectively) may be present during PSG. PSG may be normal.
5. MSLT: Normal daytime SOL.
6. Key points:
    a. Unlike adjustment sleep disorder (i.e., acute sleep disturbance that is related to an identifiable precipitating factor), psychophysiologic insomnia persists even after resolution of the inciting stressor/s.
    b. Unlike generalized anxiety disorder (i.e., anxiety is present in several aspects of daily living), anxiety in psychophysiologic insomnia is limited to issues related to sleep.

Common medications that can cause insomnia
1. Antidepressants (e.g., fluoxetine or protriptyline).
2. β-Blockers.
3. Bronchodilators.
4. Decongestants.
5. Steroids.
6. Stimulants.

Summary of causes of insomnia

I once met a man who claimed to have never slept.
> *And to prove his point,*
> *he shared with me a diary that he had kept.*
There it was – night after night of sleepless activity it seems:
> *Cooking and reading and mopping;*
> *he even went to the gym.*
He did so much from his nightly chores, he stated
> *He had nothing left to do in the day but go to bed.*
He would put on his pajamas at the crack of dawn
> *And close his eyes till two past noon.*
The first thing he'll do the minute he got out of bed
> *Is to make a list of things to do for the night ahead.*

Diagnoses: Paradoxical insomnia, delayed sleep phase syndrome and inadequate sleep hygiene.

Evaluation of insomnia
1. History and sleep diary.
2. Psychometric tests (for selected patients).
3. PSG, actigraphy and laboratory tests are not routinely indicated. PSG may be considered for insomnia suspected to be due to SRBD, PLMD or paradoxical insomnia.

PSG features of insomnia
1. ↑ SOL, ↓ SE, ↓ TST and ↑ WASO.
2. ↓ N3 and ↓ R (in some).
3. ↑ High-frequency beta (14-45 Hz) activity (quantitative EEG).
4. ↑ SOL (MSLT).
5. Note: PSG may be normal.

Therapy of insomnia
1. Goals of therapy:
    a. Alleviation of nighttime sleep disturbance.
    b. Relief of daytime consequences.
2. Types of therapy:
    a. General measures (including sleep hygiene).
    b. Non-pharmacologic therapy.

c. Pharmacologic agents.

General measures
1. Address factors that can precipitate or perpetuate sleep disturbance.
2. Identify and treat comorbid causes of insomnia (e.g., OSA, RLS or mood disorder).
3. Referral to a sleep clinician specializing in the treatment of insomnia for cases of intractable or atypical sleep disturbance.

Sleep hygiene
1. A necessary component of therapy for insomnia, but is rarely sufficiently effective, by itself, to reverse sleep disturbance.
2. Encourage bedtime activities and behaviors that enhance sleep propensity.
   a. Regular bedtime and waking time.
3. Eliminate activities and behaviors that curtail sleep propensity.
   a. Prolonged naps during the day, especially in the late afternoon and early evening.
   b. Spending excessive time awake in bed.
   c. Ingestion of alcohol and caffeine close to bedtime.
   d. Smoking close to bedtime.
   e. Using medications that can cause insomnia.
   f. Stimulating activities late in the evening.
   g. Environmental factors that interfere with sleep onset and continuity (e.g., bright lights or excessive noise).
   h. Use of bed and bedroom for non-sleep-related activities.

Cognitive-behavioral treatments for insomnia
1. First-line therapy for chronic insomnia (both primary and comorbid).
2. Types of techniques:
   a. Cognitive therapy.
   b. Paradoxical intention.
   c. Relaxation techniques.
   d. Sleep restriction.
   e. Stimulus control.
3. Improves sleep in both primary and comorbid insomnia.
4. Benefits of non-pharmacologic treatments for insomnia:
   a. ↓ Subjective symptoms of sleep disturbance. ↑ Subjective sleep quality.
   b. ↓ Use of hypnotic medications. ↓ Healthcare utilization.
   c. ↓ SOL (more effective than pharmacotherapy).
   d. ↓ WASO.
   e. ↑ TST (less effective than pharmacotherapy).
   f. ↑ SE.
   g. Note: Subjective reports of improvements in sleep are generally greater than objective measures obtained with PSG.
5. Most effective of the non-pharmacologic treatments for insomnia:
   a. Sleep restriction.
   b. Stimulus control.
6. Short-term benefits are comparable to pharmacologic therapy. Unlike pharmacotherapy, beneficial effects are sustained over time after the initial treatment period. At long-term follow-up, CBT was more effective than pharmacotherapy. However, combination CBT *plus* pharmacologic treatment is associated with *worse* outcomes than CBT alone.

Cognitive therapy
1. Addresses dysfunctional beliefs (inappropriate expectations and excessive worry) accompanying insomnia.
2. Techniques include *decatastrophization, cognitive restructuring, attention shifting* and *reappraisal* that identify irrational cognitive processes, challenges unrealistic concerns, and provide a more appropriate understanding of sleep disturbance and daytime impairment.

Paradoxical intention
1. Designed to decrease performance anxiety associated with efforts to fall asleep.
2. The technique:
   a. "Go to bed at night and to try to stay awake as long as you can."

Relaxation techniques
1. Reduction of somatic and cognitive hyperarousal.
2. Techniques:
   a. Progressive muscle relaxation (for somatic arousal; sequential tensing and relaxing various muscle groups throughout the body).
   b. Biofeedback (for somatic arousal).
   c. Guided imagery (for cognitive arousal).

Sleep restriction
1. Increasing homeostatic sleep drive (due to sleep deprivation) by reducing time in bed.

Time in bed is subsequently increased once sleep efficiency improves.
2. The technique:
   a. "Maintain a daily sleep log."
   b. "Limit time spent in bed to actual sleep time only (at least 4.5-5 hours per night)."
   c. "Advance or delay bedtime based on calculated sleep efficiency ([total sleep time/time in bed] X 100%) for the prior 5 nights until the desired sleep duration is reached".
   d. "Advance bedtime by 15-30 minutes if sleep efficiency is greater than 90%."
   e. "Delay bedtime by 15-30 minutes if sleep efficiency is less than 80%."
   f. "Do not change bedtime if sleep efficiency is between 80% and 90%."
   g. "Wake up at the same time every morning."
   h. "Do not nap during the day."

Summary:
1. *If SE > 90%: Earlier bedtime.*
2. *If SE 80-90%: Same bedtime.*
3. *If SE < 80%: Later bedtime.*

Stimulus control
1. Designed to strengthen the association of the bedroom and bedtime to a conditioned response for sleep.
2. Useful for both sleep-onset and sleep-maintenance insomnia.
3. Benefits: ↓ SOL and ↓ WASO.
4. The technique:
   a. "Use the bed only for sleep or sex."
   b. "Lie down to sleep only when sleepy."
   c. "If unable to fall asleep (within approximately 10-20 minutes), get out of bed and go to another room. Engage in a restful activity, and return to bed only when sleepy."
   d. "Wake up at the same time every morning."
   e. "Do not nap during the day."

Multi-component cognitive behavioral therapy
1. Treatment that commonly includes sleep hygiene, cognitive therapy, relaxation techniques, sleep restriction and stimulus control.

Review of cognitive-behavioral treatments for insomnia
1. Avoid alcohol – *"You might feel good, but you will feel worse."*
2. Cognitive therapy – *"Many of the things you think you know about your sleep are wrong."*
3. Paradoxical intention - *"I dare you to try to stay awake."*
4. Relaxation techniques - *"Relax. Relax. Relax."*
5. Sleep restriction – *"Less bedtime for more sleep time."*
6. Stimulus control – *"Do not multi-task in bed."*
7. Multi-component cognitive behavioral therapy – *"Let's try everything."*

Pharmacotherapy of insomnia
1. Ramelteon and zaleplon for sleep-onset insomnia.
2. BZ, eszopiclone and zolpidem for sleep-onset and sleep-maintenance insomnia.
3. Insufficient evidence regarding the efficacy of sedating antidepressants, antipsychotic agents, antihistamines and botanical compounds for the treatment of insomnia.
4. PSG effects of hypnotic agents: ↓ SOL, ↑ SE, ↑ TST and ↓ WASO.
   a. BZ: ↑ N2 (more sleep spindles), ↓ N3 and ↓ R.
5. *Important reminders:*
   a. Hypnotic agents may enhance sleep but they do not necessarily improve daytime performance.
   b. There is minimal long-term beneficial effects on sleep following discontinuation of hypnotic agents.

Indications for hypnotic agents
1. Transient sleep disruption (e.g., jet lag or adjustment sleep disorder).
2. Chronic primary insomnia that fails to respond to CBT.
3. Chronic comorbid insomnia that does not improve with treatment of the underlying condition and CBT.

Characteristics of hypnotic agents
1. Onset of action is affected by (1) rate of drug absorption (Tmax or time to peak plasma concentration) and (2) rate of distribution in the CNS. Onset of action of a drug influences sleep latency.
2. Duration of action is affected by (1) dose administered, (2) elimination half-life and (3) rate of metabolism *(greater dose, longer*

half-life and lower rate of metabolism results in longer duration of action). Duration of action of a drug influences sleep maintenance.
   a. Drugs with half-lives > 4 hours are required for therapy of sleep maintenance insomnia.
3. Potency of action is determined by (1) dose administered and (2) receptor affinity.

Elimination half-lives of hypnotic agents
1. Less than 1 hour:
   a. Ramelteon.
   b. Zaleplon.
2. 2 to 5 hours:
   a. Eszopiclone.
   b. Triazolam.
   c. Zolpidem.
3. 5 to 24 hours:
   a. Estazolam.
   b. Temazepam.
4. Greater than 40 hours:
   a. Flurazepam.
   b. Quazepam.

Selection of hypnotic agents based on timing of insomnia
1. Short-acting agents for sleep-onset insomnia.
2. Intermediate-acting agents for concurrent sleep-onset and sleep-maintenance insomnia.
3. Long-acting agents for early morning awakenings and daytime anxiety.

Benzodiazepines and non-benzodiazepine benzodiazepine receptor agonists
1. Bind to the gamma-aminobutyric acid-benzodiazepine (GABA-BZ) receptor complex.
   a. The GABA-A receptor consists of 5 subunits, typically 2 alpha, 2 beta and 1 gamma subunit. The BZ receptor is located at the interface between an alpha and gamma subunit.
   b. Attachment of GABA, an inhibitory neurotransmitter, to the GABA-A receptor causes the chloride channel to open, leading to an influx of ions into the cell and hyperpolarization. This inhibitory response is enhanced (positive allosteric modulation) when BZ receptor agonists attach to the BZ site (i.e., greater influx of chloride ions).
2. Various GABA-BZ receptor subunits have different actions.

   a. BZ1: Hypnotic and amnesic actions.
   b. BZ2 and BZ3: Muscle relaxation, anti-seizure and anti-anxiety actions.

Benzodiazepines
1. Bind non-selectively to the different GABA-BZ receptor subunits, BZ1, BZ2 and BZ3.
2. In addition to their hypnotic properties, they are also potent anxiolytics, myorelaxants and anticonvulsants.

Adverse effects of benzodiazepines
1. Rebound daytime anxiety (with short-acting agents).
2. Daytime sleepiness (with long-acting agents).
3. Cognitive and psychomotor impairment (motor incoordination, delayed reaction time, confusion and amnesia).
4. Development of tolerance (need for increasingly higher dosages to attain similar therapeutic benefit during chronic use).
5. Withdrawal symptoms (anxiety, irritability and restlessness).
6. Dependency and abuse liability (low risk).
7. Relapse (recurrence of insomnia following drug discontinuation).
8. Rebound insomnia (worsening of sleep disturbance compared to pretreatment levels after drug discontinuation; more likely to occur with long-term use of short-acting and intermediate-acting agents).
9. Respiratory depression and worsening of OSA.
10. Increase in falls (in some older adults).

Contraindications to benzodiazepine use
1. Pregnancy and lactation.
2. Significant renal or hepatic impairment (requires dosage adjustment).
3. Untreated OSA.
4. Severe obstructive and restrictive ventilatory impairment.

Non-benzodiazepine benzodiazepine receptor agonists
1. Selectively bind to the BZ1 receptor subunit.
2. Duration of action (shortest to longest): zaleplon < zolpidem < eszopiclone.
3. Compared to conventional benzodiazepines:
   a. Similar hypnotic action.
   b. No muscle relaxant, anticonvulsant or anxiolytic properties.
   c. Less likely to cause rebound insomnia, withdrawal symptoms or tolerance.
   d. Less likely to alter sleep architecture.

    e.   Minimal abuse or addiction liability.
    f.   No active metabolites.
4. FDA Schedule IV controlled substances.

Melatonin receptor agonist

1. Ramelteon.
2. Selective agonist for the SCN melatonin receptor subtypes, MT1 (attenuation of arousal) and MT2 (phase shifting of circadian rhythms).
3. Short half-life. Indicated for sleep-onset insomnia.
4. Contraindications: Use of fluvoxamine and hepatic impairment.

Sedating antidepressants and antipsychotic agents

1. Limited published data on their appropriate use for insomnia. Not recommended for the treatment of insomnia.
2. Trazodone.
   a. No significant potential for tolerance or dependency.
   b. Possible adverse effects include cardiac arrhythmias, orthostatic hypotension and priapism.
   c. Can give rise to serotonin syndrome when administered with other serotonin-specific agents.
3. Nefazodone.
   a. Associated with rare liver toxicity.
4. Mirtazapine.
5. Tricyclic antidepressants (sedating).
   a. Amitriptyline, doxepin, nortriptyline and trimipramine.
   b. Adverse effects include anti-cholinergic actions (e.g., urinary retention or constipation), cardiac arrhythmias, orthostatic hypotension, and exacerbation of RLS and PLMD.

6. Sedating antipsychotic agents (e.g., quetiapine and olanzapine).

Non-prescription hypnotic agents

1. Not recommended for the treatment of insomnia. Limited published data on their efficacy as sleep aids for insomnia.
2. First generation histamine antagonists (e.g., diphenhydramine).
   a. Sedating.
   b. PSG effects: $\downarrow$ SOL and $\uparrow$ TST.
   c. Constitute the majority of over-the-counter hypnotic agents.
   d. Second-generation agents (e.g., loratadine and fexofenadine) are less likely to cause sedation.
   e. Adverse effects of histamine antagonists:
      i. Rapid development of tolerance to hypnotic effect.
      ii. Residual daytime sedation because of long half-lives.
      iii. Anti-cholinergic effects: Confusion, delirium, dizziness, blurring of vision, dry mouth, urinary retention, constipation and $\uparrow$ intraocular pressure in narrow angle glaucoma.
3. Melatonin.
   a. Used primarily for treating insomnia associated with CRSDs.
   b. Not FDA-approved for the therapy of insomnia.
   c. Short half-life of 20-30 minutes.
4. Botanical compounds.
   a. There is inconclusive evidence for the efficacy of kava, passionflower, skullcap or valerian as treatment for insomnia.
   b. Hepatotoxicity has been described with kava and valerian.

Sleepy Days

In this section
General
Behaviorally-induced insufficient sleep syndrome
Idiopathic hypersomnia
Recurrent hypersomnia
Hypersomnia due to medical, neurological or psychiatric disorders
Hypersomnia due to drugs or substance
Evaluation of EDS
Effective countermeasures for EDS

General
1. Excessive sleepiness is defined as an inability to consistently achieve and sustain wakefulness and alertness to accomplish the tasks of daily living.
2. EDS can manifest as frequent napping, sleep attacks or microsleep episodes. EDS can also present as hyperactivity in children or as automatic behavior.
3. Prevalence is greater among adolescents and older adults. Gender: M = F.
4. Consequences of EDS include:
   a. ↑ Risk of accidents.
   b. ↑ Absenteeism.
   c. ↓ Work and academic performance.
   d. Mood disorder.
5. General causes of EDS:
   a. Inadequate sleep duration.
   b. Sleep fragmentation.
   c. Disorders of the CNS sleep-wake apparatus.
   d. Disturbance of circadian rhythm timing of sleep and waking.
   e. Medication and substance use or withdrawal.

Behaviorally-induced insufficient sleep syndrome
1. EDS is due to chronic voluntary, but unintentional, SD. Improvement in symptoms occurs following longer sleep duration (such as during weekends or holidays).
2. This is the most common cause of EDS.
3. Increased prevalence among adolescents. Gender: M > F.
4. Diagnosis is based on clinical history and sleep diaries. PSG is not indicated.
5. PSG and MSLT features:
   a. PSG: ↓ SOL, ↑ SE, ↑ TST (when sleep is permitted to continue *ad lib*), ↓ WASO, ↑ N3 and ↑ R.
   b. MSLT: ↓ SOL (< 8 minutes +/-

SOREMPs).
6. Therapy involves sleep extension.

Idiopathic hypersomnia
1. Constant sleepiness despite sufficient, or even increased, amounts of nighttime sleep and daytime napping. No identifiable cause.
2. Compared to narcolepsy, naps are longer and less refreshing. No cataplexy.
3. Associated clinical features: Automatic behavior, confusion upon awakening, disorientation, headaches, orthostatic hypotension, Reynaud's-type vascular symptoms and syncope.
4. Classified as either: (a) *with long sleep time* [nocturnal sleep ≥ 10 h and ≥ 1 daytime nap of > 1 hour], or (b) *without long sleep time* [nocturnal sleep > 6 but < 10 hours].
5. Gender: M = F. Onset commonly during adolescence or early adulthood. Course is typically chronic.
6. Diagnosis requires PSG and MSLT. Monitoring esophageal pressures to exclude UARS is recommended. Normal CSF hypocretin-1 levels. Neurological examination is usually normal.
   a. PSG features: ↓ SOL, ↑ SE, ↑ or normal TST, ↓ WASO, ↑ N3 (in some) and no change in REM SL.
   b. MSLT: ↓ Mean SOL (< 8 [6 +/- 3] minutes) and < 2 SOREMPs.
7. Therapy consists of sleep hygiene and stimulant agents (however, less favorable and les predictable response to stimulants compared to narcolepsy).

Recurrent hypersomnia
1. Recurrent episodes of EDS that occur weeks or months apart, typically about 10 times annually.
2. Normal sleep, alertness and general behavior between episodes.
3. Either monosymptomatic (sleepiness only,

such as menstrual-related hypersomnia) or polysymptomatic/Kleine Levin syndrome (sleepiness, hyperphagia, hypersexuality, aggressiveness, abnormal behavior and cognitive impairment).

  a. Menstrual-related hypersomnia:
    i. EDS lasts about 1 week with rapid resolution of symptoms at the time of menses. Use of oral contraceptives leads to prolonged remission.
  b. Kleine-Levin syndrome:
    i. *Useful mnemonic is SEXY:*
        Sleepiness.
        Eating.
        Xtacy.
        Young men.

4. Rare. Gender: M > F (Kleine-Levin syndrome). M = F (monosymptomatic type).
5. Onset during early adolescence. Severity of hypersomnia may decrease over time in Kleine-Levin syndrome.
6. Unknown etiology. Diencephalic hypoperfusion in SPECT scan in Kleine-Levin syndrome.
7. PSG: ↓ SE and ↑ WASO.
8. 24-hour PSG: ↑ TST (≥ 18 hours).
9. Consider trial of lithium therapy in Kleine-Levin syndrome.

Hypersomnia due to medical, neurological or psychiatric disorders
1. Sufficient nighttime sleep duration (> 6 hours). Cataplexy is absent.
2. Medical disorders that can cause hypersomnia:
  a. Hepatic encephalopathy.
  b. Hypothyroidism.
  c. Niemann Pick type C disease.
  d. Prader-Willi syndrome.
  e. Renal failure.
3. Neurological disorders that can cause hypersomnia:
  a. CNS infections or tumor.
  b. Head trauma.
  c. Parkinson disease.
  d. Stroke.
4. Psychiatric disorders that can cause hypersomnia:
  a. Atypical depression.
  b. Bipolar type II mood disorder.
  c. Seasonal affective disorder.

Hypersomnia due to drugs or substance
1. Use or abuse of sedative-hypnotic agents.
2. Withdrawal from stimulant agents.

Evaluation of EDS
1. Sleep history. Sleep diary +/- actigraphy.
2. Subjective tests of sleepiness (e.g., ESS and Stanford sleepiness scale).
3. Severity of sleepiness based on ESS: Aggregate score: 0-9 (normal), ≥ 10 (sleepiness present; advice from a sleep specialist recommended).
4. PSG (to exclude OSA and PLMD).
5. MSLT.
  a. Sleepiness is defined by a mean SOL < 8 minutes.
  b. Mean+/- SD sleep latencies:
    i. 10 +/- 4 minutes in healthy persons.
    ii. 3 +/- 3 minutes for narcolepsy.
    iii. 6 +/- 3 minutes for idiopathic hypersomnia.
6. MWT.
  a. SOL < 40 minutes.

Effective countermeasures for EDS
1. Sleep extension (for insufficient sleep syndrome).
2. Napping.
  a. Long naps (e.g., > 2 hours) may cause sleep inertia.
3. Bright light therapy for SWSD and jet lag.
4. Caffeine: Caffeine and napping have additive effects.
5. Stimulant agents: Amphetamines, methylphenidate or modafinil.

Narcolepsy

General

1. A neurological disorder characterized by the clinical tetrad of EDS and manifestations of REM sleep physiology during wakefulness (e.g., cataplexy, sleep paralysis and sleep hallucinations).
   a. Only about 10-15% of persons with narcolepsy demonstrate this full tetrad.
2. *A useful mnemonic for narcolepsy is CHIPS:*
   Think orexin (appetite) ⇒ chips.
      Cataplexy.
      Hallucinations.
      Insomnia (sleep disturbance).
      Paralysis.
      Sleepiness.
3. Prevalence of clinical features:
   a. EDS: ≈ 100%.
   b. Cataplexy: ≈ 60-90%.
   c. Sleep paralysis: ≈ 5-65%.
   d. Sleep hallucinations: ≈ 8-70%.
   e. Sleep disturbance: 50-80%.
   f. Automatic behavior: 8-40%.

Excessive sleepiness

1. Generally the first, primary and most disabling symptom of narcolepsy.
2. Brief naps, usually lasting 10-20 minutes, occur repeatedly throughout the day. EDS transiently improves after awakening from a nap but gradually increases within 2-3 hours.
   a. The repetitive short naps seen in adults contrast with the prolonged sleep periods in children.
3. *Sleep attacks* - Sudden, irresistible episodes of sleepiness that occur abruptly without warning leading to sleep during inappropriate places or circumstances.

Cataplexy

1. Abrupt and transient episodes of muscle atonia or hypotonia during wakefulness that are typically precipitated by intense emotion (e.g., laughter, anger or excitement).
   a. Cataplexy may also be triggered during the switch to modafinil from amphetamines.
2. Recovery is immediate and complete, but prolonged episodes may give rise to REM

sleep.
3. Generally < 2 minutes in duration.
4. Most commonly affected areas are the lower extremities, face, jaw and neck.
   a. Respiratory and oculomotor muscles are spared.
   b. Blurring of vision may occur.
5. Memory and consciousness are unaffected.
6. Commonly occurs 1-3 times weekly (variable). Frequency of cataplexy may decrease over time.
7. Physical examination during an episode of cataplexy may demonstrate muscle flaccidity, reduction or absence of deep tendon reflexes, and a positive Babinski sign.
8. Note:
   a. Cataplexy is the only pathognomonic symptom of narcolepsy. Nevertheless, the absence of cataplexy does not exclude a diagnosis of narcolepsy.
   b. *Status cataplecticus*: Repetitive episodes of cataplexy occurring in succession that may develop following withdrawal of REM sleep suppressant agents.

Sleep hallucinations
1. Hallucinatory phenomena may be visual, auditory, tactile or kinetic.
2. Occur during wakefulness at sleep onset (hypnagogic) or upon awakening (hypnopompic).
3. May be accompanied by sleep paralysis.
4. Not pathognomonic for narcolepsy. Recurrent sleep hallucinations are present in about 4% of healthy individuals.

Sleep paralysis
1. Transient muscle paralysis occurs either at sleep onset (hypnagogic) or upon awakening (hypnopompic). Duration of a few seconds or minutes.
2. Affects voluntary muscles with sparing of respiratory, oculomotor and sphincter muscles.
3. Sensorium is unaffected.
4. Recovery is immediate and complete.

Sleep disturbance
1. Poor sleep quality with repetitive arousals and awakenings.
2. Affected persons may complain of sleep-maintenance insomnia.

Other clinical features
1. Memory impairment.
2. Automatic behavior.
3. Visual changes - blurred vision, diplopia and ptosis.
4. Sleep drunkenness (confusion and diminished alertness immediately after an awakening).
5. Hyperactivity and learning disability (in children).

Associated disorders
1. Increased risk of developing SRBD (OSA and CSA), PLMS and RBD.
2. Increased risk of developing depression and type 2 DM.
3. High prevalence of psychopathology on the Minnesota Multiphasic Personality Inventory (MMPI).

Demographics
1. Prevalence of 0.05% in the U.S.
   a. Higher prevalence in Japan and lower prevalence in Israel.
2. Gender: M > F (narcolepsy with cataplexy).

Clinical course
1. EDS is usually the presenting symptom, followed months to years later by the emergence of cataplexy, sleep paralysis and sleep hallucinations.
2. Onset is generally during adolescence and early adulthood (15-25 years of age), and rarely before 5 years or after 60 years of age.
3. Course is typically chronic. EDS is generally persistent, whereas severity of cataplexy may decrease over time.

Pathophysiology
1. EDS is related to the loss of hypothalamic hypocretin neurons, with ↑ gliosis.
2. Also associated with:
   a. Defective cholinergic system regulating REM sleep (cholinergic supersensitivity).
   b. Defective monoaminergic regulation of cholinergic mechanisms.
   c. Impairment of dopamine system.
3. Mechanism of cataplexy:

Loss of hypocretin-induced excitation of locus ceruleus (noradrenergic) and dorsal raphe (serotonergic)
↓

Disinhibition of cholinergic neurons in LDT
and PPT nuclei
↓
Stimulation of nucleus magnocellularis
↓
Glycine-mediated hyperpolarization of the
anterior horn cells of the spinal cord

Consequences
1. Accidents.
2. Depression.
3. Obesity.
4. ↓ QOL.

Narcolepsy without cataplexy
1. Although not associated with cataplexy,
   cataplexy-like symptoms may be present
   (e.g., prolonged episodes of tiredness, or
   muscle weakness associated with atypical
   triggers, such as exercise).
2. Accounts for 10-50% of cases of narcolepsy.
3. Most persons have normal CSF hypocretin-
   1 levels.
   a. HLA DQB1*0602-negative
      narcolepsy without cataplexy
      persons generally have normal CSF
      hypocretin-1 levels.
   b. Low CSF hypocretin-1 levels are
      present in 10-20% of HLA DQB1*0602-
      positive persons with narcolepsy without
      cataplexy.
4. Loss of hypocretin-containing hypothalamic
   neurons is believed to be less severe than in
   narcolepsy with cataplexy.
5. 40% are HLA DQB1*0602 positive.

Narcolepsy secondary to medical disorders
1. Referred to as secondary narcolepsy.
2. Presence of a medical or neurological
   condition that is responsible for
   narcolepsy symptoms.
3. CSF hypocretin-1 levels are low (< 110
   pg/mL or < 1/3 of mean normal control
   values).
4. Common medical conditions causing
   narcolepsy symptoms:
   a. Hypothalamic lesions: Tumors,
      multiple sclerosis or sarcoidosis.
   b. Brainstem lesions: Degenerative,
      infectious or inflammatory.
   c. Paraneoplastic syndrome (with anti-
      Ma2 antibodies).
   d. Neiman-Pick type C disease.
   e. Head trauma.
   f. Parkinson disease.
   g. Multiple system atrophy.

h. Viral illness (unspecified).
i. Disseminated encephalomyelitis.
j. Myotonic dystrophy and Prader-Willi
   syndrome – both narcolepsy and
   SRBD.

Evaluation
1. Clinical history.
   a. Narcolepsy with cataplexy can be
      diagnosed by history alone.
2. PSG followed by MSLT is indicated when
   cataplexy is absent, atypical or equivocal.
3. Other tests of less certain diagnostic utility:
   a. Subjective scales of sleepiness, such
      as ESS or Stanford sleepiness scale.
   b. Performance vigilance testing.

Polysomnographic features
1. ↓ SOL (< 10 minutes).
2. SOREMP (REM SL ≤ 10-15 minutes) in 25-
   50% of cases.
3. ↑ N1.
4. ↑ WASO (repetitive awakenings).
5. ↓/= TST.
6. Normal R.

Multiple sleep latency test
1. Mean SOL ≤ 8 minutes (present in 90% of
   patients with narcolepsy and in 15-30% of
   normal individuals).
   a. Mean SOL: 3 +/- 3 minutes.
2. ≥ 2 SOREMPs (sensitivity: 0.7; specificity:
   0.9).
3. The combination of a shortened SOL and
   SOREMPs is present in only about 60-85%
   of cases.
4. Multiple SOREMPs are more specific for
   narcolepsy than a shortened SOL.
5. Other common causes of shortened mean
   SOL, often with SOREMPs, are SD, OSA
   and DSPD.
6. The absence of SOREMPs does not
   exclude the presence of narcolepsy, and
   their presence does not establish its
   diagnosis.

Maintenance of wakefulness test
1. May be used to monitor treatment response
   to stimulant medications used for EDS.

CSF hypocretin-1
1. CSF hypocretin-1 level ≤ 110 pg/mL or <
   1/3 of mean normal control values (in the
   absence of severe brain pathology).
   a. Highly specific and sensitive for

narcolepsy with cataplexy. A normal test does not exclude the diagnosis of narcolepsy with cataplexy (normal levels in 10% of this population).
   b. Normal levels are usually noted in narcolepsy without cataplexy.

Possible uses of CSF hypocretin-1 measurement
1. Current use of medications (e.g., stimulants or REM sleep suppressants) that may interfere with proper interpretation of MSLT results.
2. In persons who are too young to undergo MSLT.
3. Early in the disease course prior to the development of cataplexy.

HLA typing
1. Limited diagnostic utility.

Therapy: general measures
1. Proper sleep hygiene.
2. Regular sleep-wake schedules.
3. Sufficient nocturnal sleep duration.
4. Therapy of other concurrent sleep disorders that can cause EDS.
5. Avoidance of potentially dangerous activities (e.g., driving) until EDS is adequately managed.
6. Scheduled naps (seldom sufficient as sole therapy for EDS).

Treatment of excessive sleepiness
1. Armodafinil and modafinil (schedule IV drug).
2. Dextroamphetamine.
3. Methylphenidate (schedule II drug).
4. Note: Pemoline has been withdrawn from the market due to concerns regarding hepatotoxicity.

Treatment of sleep disturbance
1. Hypnotic agents.
2. γ-hydroxybutyrate (sodium oxybate).

Treatment of cataplexy, sleep paralysis and sleep hallucinations
1. REM sleep suppressant agents:
   a. SSRI: Fluoxetine.
   b. TCA:
      i. Sedating: Desipramine or imipramine.
      ii. Stimulating: Protriptyline.
   c. Non-tricyclic serotonin-norepinephrine reuptake inhibitor: Venlafaxine.
   d. MAOI.
   e. *Note*: Sudden discontinuation of REM sleep suppressants can give rise to status cataplecticus.
2. γ-hydroxybutyrate.
3. Other medications: Carbamazepine, clonidine or viloxazine.

Obstructive Sleep Apnea

General
1. Repetitive reduction or cessation of airflow, despite the presence of respiratory efforts, due to partial or complete UA occlusion during sleep.

Definitions
1. Apnea (adult): Cessation of nasal and oral airflow for ≥ 10 seconds.
   a. Central event: Respiratory efforts are absent.
   b. Obstructive event: Respiratory efforts are present.

c. Mixed event: Initial central apnea followed by obstructive apnea.
2. Hypopnea: Reduction of airflow by ≥ 30% from baseline for ≥ 10 seconds *plus* O_2 desaturation of ≥ 4%.
3. Respiratory effort related arousal (RERA): Reduction in airflow despite increasing respiratory effort (progressively more negative esophageal pressures) for ≥ 10 seconds that ends with an arousal. Not associated with significant O_2 desaturation (< 4% fall in SaO_2).

4. Complex sleep apnea: Central apneas develop or become more frequent during CPAP titration for OSA.
5. Apnea hypopnea index: Sum of apneas and hypopneas per hour of sleep.

Classification of severity based on AHI
1. *Mild*: 5-15.
2. *Moderate*: 16-30.
3. *Severe*: > 30.
Note: Other factors that influence the clinical severity of OSA include (a) degree of EDS, (b) nadir of SaO_2, (c) extent of sleep fragmentation, (d) presence of nocturnal arrhythmias and (e) co-morbid cardiovascular or neurological disorders.

Etiology of night-to-night variability of AHI in persons with OSA
1. Changes in % REM sleep.
2. Changes in percentage of supine vs. non-supine sleep.
3. Changes in nasal resistance (e.g., congestion).
4. Use of alcohol, muscle relaxants, sedatives or opioids.
5. Change in weight (over time).

Demographics
1. Prevalence:
   a. 24% of adult men and 9% of adult women (if OSA is defined by an AHI of ≥ 5).
   b. 4% of adult men and 2% of adult women (if OSA is defined by an AHI ≥ 5 *plus* complaints of EDS).
   c. More common in children (ages 3-5 years) than adolescents.
   d. 30-80% of older adults.
2. Gender: M > F. Prevalence increases in women with menopause.

The upper airway as a collapsible cylinder
1. UA airflow is determined by (a) the difference between upstream (i.e., nasal) and downstream pressure, and (b) airway resistance. Thus, airflow is greater with ↑ upstream pressure, ↓ downstream pressure and ↓ airway resistance.
2. UA patency is dependent on the balance of factors that maintain airway opening (e.g., activation of dilator muscles) and those that promote airway closure (e.g., reduction in intraluminal extrathoracic airway pressure as well as Bernoulli forces). Airway size is also influenced by lung volume, both of which decrease during sleep. During wakefulness, negative intraluminal pressure triggers a reflex UA dilator muscle activation (i.e., ↑ genioglossus activity); this reflex progressively decreases during NREM and REM sleep.
3. Critical closing pressure (P_{CRIT}) is the intraluminal pressure at which the UA collapses. P_{CRIT} becomes progressively *less* negative from non-snorers and snorers to persons with OSA. Activation of UA dilator muscles decreases P_{CRIT}.

Ventilatory loop gain
1. Persons with OSA have an intrinsically unstable negative feedback ventilatory control system. This high ventilatory loop gain increases the likelihood of periodic breathing even in cases of minimal respiratory perturbations.

Pathophysiology of OSA
1. Compared to controls, persons with OSA tend to have narrower UA that are more vulnerable to collapse. The most common sites of UA obstruction are retropalatal (behind the palate) and retrolingual (behind the tongue).
2. Repetitive UA obstruction due to reduced activity of UA dilating muscles during sleep is associated with:
   a. Episodic falls in SaO_2.
   b. Snoring (alternating with periods of silence).
   c. Arrhythmias (relative bradycardia during airway obstruction followed by tachycardia during termination of apnea).
   d. Arousal at the termination of the event.
   e. ↑ BP in the immediate post-apneic period.

Factors increasing severity of oxygen desaturation in OSA
1. ↓ Awake supine SaO_2.
2. ↓ Baseline sleep SaO_2.
3. ↑ % of TST with apneas or hypopneas.
4. ↑ Duration of apnea or hypopneas.
5. ↓ Duration of normal ventilation between periods of apnea or hypopnea.

6. ↓ FRC and ERV.
7. Presence of comorbid lung disorders (e.g., COPD).
8. Stage of sleep (more severe during REM than NREM sleep).
9. Type of apnea (more severe with obstructive than central apneas).

Risk factors for OSA
1. *+ Family history of OSA.*
2. *Male gender* (for adults): M:F ratio of 2-3:1.
3. *Menopausal state in women*: Postmenopausal women using HRT have less risk of OSA than nonusers (in some studies).
4. *Aging*: Increase in risk up to middle age (50-55 years of age).
5. *Excess body weight*: Major risk factor. A 10% increase in weight is associated with a 6-fold increase in risk for OSA. Central obesity (waist-hip ratio) is more important than general obesity.
6. *Snoring.*
7. *Specific cranio-facial and oropharyngeal features*, including:
   a. Increasing neck circumference (> 17 inches in men and > 16 inches in women).
   b. Nasal narrowing or congestion.
   c. Macroglossia.
   d. Low-lying soft palate.
   e. Enlarged tonsils and adenoids (especially in children).
   f. Mid-face hypoplasia, retrognathia, micrognathia or mandibular hypoplasia.
   g. Tracheal stenosis and laryngomalacia.
8. *Hereditary syndromes*:
   a. Maxillary hypoplasia:
      i. Antley-Bixler.
      ii. Apert.
      iii. Crouzon.
      iv. Down.
      v. Pfeiffer.
      vi. Stickler.
   b. Mandibular hypoplasia:
      i. Goldenhar.
      ii. Pierre-Robin.
      iii. Treacher Collins.
   c. Tongue enlargement:
      i. Beckwith-Wiedeman.
      ii. Hunter.
   d. Notes: The degree of craniofacial disfigurement may not correlate with OSA severity. Routine screening for OSA is recommended for persons with craniofacial syndromes.

9. *Race* (African-Americans, Mexican-Americans, Asians and Pacific Islanders).
10. *Smoking and alcohol use.*
11. *Medications* (e.g., muscle relaxants, sedatives, anesthetics and opioid analgesics). NBBRAs do not significantly affect AHI.
12. *Primary disorders* (e.g., untreated hypothyroidism [inconsistent data], acromegaly, androgen therapy, amyloidosis, CHF, narcolepsy, neuromuscular disorders, polycystic ovarian syndrome and stroke).

Common clinical features of OSA
1. Daytime sleepiness (most common complaint).
   a. Severity of EDS does not correlate closely with AHI.
2. Attention deficit and/or hyperactivity (in children).
3. Changes in mood (particularly treatment-resistant depression).
4. Decline in performance at work or school.
5. Dry mouth/throat sensation upon awakening.
6. Fatigue.
7. Gastroesophageal reflux.
8. Impaired cognition (memory and concentration).
9. Insomnia.
10. Morning headaches.
11. Nighttime diaphoresis.
12. Nocturia.
13. Nonrestorative or unrefreshing sleep or naps.
14. Repeated awakenings with gasping or choking.
15. Snoring.
16. Witnessed apneas.

Common physical findings in persons with OSA
1. Crowded posterior pharyngeal space.
2. Dental malocclusion.
3. Enlarged tonsils and adenoids; prominent tonsillar pillars (especially among children).
4. Excess body weight (BMI > 25).
5. High, narrow hard palate.
6. Large neck circumference.
7. Large uvula.
8. Low-lying soft palate.
9. Macroglossia.
10. Narrow oropharynx (maxilla and mandible).
11. Nasal septal deviation or turbinate hypertrophy.
12. Retro- or micrognathia.

Note: Physical examination may be entirely unremarkable.

Common associated features of OSA
1. Cardiac arrhythmias.
2. Congestive heart failure.
3. Insulin resistance.
4. Ischemic heart disease.
5. Nocturnal seizures.
6. Parasomnias (e.g., confusional arousals and sleep-related eating disorder).
7. Pulmonary hypertension and cor pulmonale (in severe OSA).
8. Sleep bruxism.
9. Systemic hypertension.

Consequences of untreated OSA
1. ↑ Mortality (among young and middle-age adults).
2. ↑ Driving and work-related accidents (especially in sleepy persons).
3. Negative impact on school and work performance.
4. ↓ SaO_2 and PaO_2, and ↑ $PaCO_2$ during sleep.
5. ↑ Systemic and pulmonary artery pressure. ↓ LV and RV output. ↑ PVR.
6. Neurocognitive and psychiatric effects:
   a. Depression and anxiety. "Irritable" mood.
   b. ↓ QOL.
   c. ↓ Alertness and vigilance.
   d. Impairment of neurocognitive performance (executive function, learning and memory).
7. Sleep disturbance. EDS and/or insomnia. Extent of sleep fragmentation, rather than AHI, correlates better with severity of EDS.
8. Cardiovascular effects:
   a. Systemic hypertension (independent of obesity).
      i. Each additional apnea event per hour of sleep increases the odds of hypertension by about 1%.
      ii. Each 10% decrease in nocturnal SaO_2 increases the odds of hypertension by 13%.
      iii. Failure of systemic BP to fall during sleep ("non-dipping").
      iv. Prevalence of OSA is increased in persons with drug-resistant hypertension.
      v. Treatment of OSA may decrease BP and improve hypertension control.
   b. Pulmonary hypertension and cor pulmonale.
      i. Degree of O_2 desaturation may be predictive of the development of pulmonary hypertension.
      ii. ↑ Likelihood in persons with daytime hypoxemia and hypercapnia, morbid obesity, or underlying COPD.
      iii. Degree of pulmonary hypertension is generally mild and lower than that in primary pulmonary hypertension.
      iv. PAP therapy can improve OSA-related pulmonary hypertension.
   c. Coronary artery disease.
   d. Congestive heart failure.
      i. ↑ Prevalence of OSA in persons with CHF. OSA, in turn, can worsen heart function.
   e. Cardiac arrhythmias.
      i. Sinus arrhythmia [most common].
      ii. Other arrhythmias: Atrioventricular block, bradycardia, premature ventricular contractions, sinus pause and ventricular tachycardia.
      iii. ↑ Likelihood of recurrence of atrial fibrillation after successful cardioversion in untreated OSA.
   f. Cerebrovascular disease.
      i. ↑ Risk of strokes in persons with OSA.
      ii. ↑ Risk of OSA following strokes.
9. Miscellaneous consequences:
   a. Erectile dysfunction.
   b. Gastroesophageal reflux.
   c. Insulin resistance.
   d. Nocturia.
   e. ↑ Healthcare utilization.

Causes of neurocognitive impairment in OSA
1. Sleep fragmentation.
2. Sleep-related hypoxemia giving rise to neuronal injury.

Evaluation of OSA
1. Clinical history.
2. Physical examination.
3. Laboratory testing.
   a. Routine screening for hypothyroidism is *not* indicated unless other clinical features suggestive of hypothyroidism are present.
4. PSG is required for the diagnosis of OSA. Neither clinical nor physical examination features are sufficiently sensitive or specific for OSA. The current standard of practice is an attended laboratory study with technologist-attended PAP titration using either full-night (with separate diagnostic and PAP titration studies) or split-night (consisting of an initial diagnostic portion and a subsequent PAP titration on the same night) protocols.
   a. PSG features: ↑ WASO, ↑ N1, ↑ N2, ↓ N3 and ↓ R.
   b. Respiratory events are generally more frequent, last longer, and are associated with more profound O_2 desaturation during REM sleep compared to NREM sleep.
   c. Paradoxical breathing ("out-of-phase" motion of the ribcage and abdomen).
   d. Large inspiratory and expiratory pressure swings during esophageal manometry.
   e. ↑ Pulse transit time (PTT; duration for the arterial pulse pressure wave to travel from the aortic valve to the periphery) during OSA-related inspiratory fall in BP. ↓ PTT during arousal-related rise in BP.
5. *MSLT* is indicated if EDS persists despite optimal PAP therapy.
6. *UA imaging studies* (lateral cephalometric views, CT or MRI of the UA) may be considered for patients with craniofacial syndromes, especially prior to surgical therapy.

Effect of REM sleep (compared to NREM sleep) on OSA
1. ↓ UA dilating muscle activity.
2. ↓ Lung volumes.
3. ↓ Hypoxic and hypercapnic ventilatory drive.
4. ↑ Duration of apnea-hypopnea events.
5. ↑ O_2 desaturation related to apnea-hypopneas.

Therapy of OSA
1. General measures.
2. Positive airway pressure therapy.
3. Oral devices.
4. UA surgery.

General measures
1. Avoidance of alcohol, BZ, opioids and muscle relaxants that can decrease UA muscle activity.
2. Avoidance of smoking.
3. Sleep hygiene. Avoidance of SD.
4. Safety counseling (i.e., avoidance of driving whenever drowsy).
5. Optimal weight management. Regular exercise.
6. Positional therapy: Avoidance of a supine sleep position in persons whose respiratory events occur exclusively or predominantly during a supine sleep position and in whom PSG demonstrates a normal AHI in the lateral or prone sleep position. Requires regular follow-up.
7. O_2 therapy (not indicated as sole therapy for OSA). It may be considered for persons with significant nocturnal hypoxemia that is not controlled by PAP therapy alone.
8. Nasal dilators are not sufficiently effective when used alone to treat OSA.
9. Pharmacologic treatment.
   a. Topical nasal corticosteroids may be a useful adjunct to primary therapies for OSA in persons with concurrent rhinitis.
   b. Thyroid hormone replacement for hypothyroid states. Restoration of the euthyroid state does not completely abolish apnea and hypopneas in every hypothyroid person with OSA. Angina can develop in persons with ischemic heart disease and untreated OSA during thyroid hormone replacement therapy.
   c. Hormone replacement therapy for postmenopausal women (efficacy data are conflicting).
   d. Modafinil and armodafinil are recommended for treating residual EDS in persons on effective PAP therapy and with no other known cause for EDS.

Summary:
1. *Positional therapy for OSA - "Get off your back."*
2. *Weight control for obesity and OSA - Fat is bad.*
3. *Pharmacologic therapy for OSA: Most don't work.*

Positive airway pressure therapy
1. Treatment of choice for most persons with OSA.
2. Mechanism of action:
   a. Functions as a pneumatic splint that maintains UA patency. PAP increases intraluminal UA pressure above P_{CRIT}.
   b. Higher pressures may be required to control respiratory events during REM sleep and supine sleep.

Indications for PAP therapy
1. AHI of ≥ 15 events per hour; or
2. AHI of ≥ 5 and ≤ 14 events per hour *plus* complaints of EDS, impaired cognition, mood disorder or insomnia, *or* documented HTN or CAD, *or* history of stroke.
3. Note: AHI should be based on ≥ 2 hours of PSG-recorded sleep.

Positive airway pressure modalities
1. *Continuous positive airway pressure* (CPAP): A single constant pressure is provided throughout the respiratory cycle.
2. *CPAP with expiratory pressure relief technology* (Cflex): A single pressure is provided but allows for a transient reduction in pressure during expiration and a subsequent return of pressure to baseline setting before initiation of the next inspiration.
3. *Bi-level positive airway pressure* (BPAP): Two pressure levels are provided during the respiratory cycle, namely a higher level during inspiration (inspiratory positive airway pressure [IPAP]) and a lower pressure during expiration (expiratory positive airway pressure [EPAP]).
4. *Auto-titrating positive airway pressure* (APAP): Variable pressures are provided using device-specific diagnostic and therapeutic algorithms. Automatically and continuously adjusts the delivered PAP to maintain UA patency.
5. *Adaptive servo ventilation*: Pressure support (difference between EPAP and IPAP) increases during hypoventilation and decreases during hyperventilation.
6. *Nocturnal non-invasive positive pressure ventilation:* Two pressure levels are provided at a set rate to assist ventilation.

Methods to determine optimal CPAP pressure
1. Full-night, laboratory, attended PSG (preferred method).
2. Split-night PSG.
3. APAP titration (minimal data regarding efficacy).

Criteria for split-night sleep study
1. Split-night PSG consists of an initial diagnostic portion followed by CPAP titration during the same sleep study night.
2. Requirements:
   a. ≥ 2 hours of recorded sleep time during the initial diagnostic portion of the study.
   b. AHI > 40, or 20-40 if accompanied by significant O_2 desaturation during diagnostic portion of the study.
   c. ≥ 3 hours available for adequate CPAP titration with the documentation of REM sleep during supine sleep.

Beneficial effects of PAP therapy for OSA
1. ↓ Mortality (reversal of the increase in mortality associated with OSA).
2. ↓ Sleepiness (subjective and objective).
3. ↑ Sleep quality (inconsistent). ↓ Frequency of arousals.
4. ↓ Snoring. ↓ AHI. ↑ SaO_2.
5. ↑ QOL (inconclusive data).
6. ↑ Neurocognitive function (inconsistent data). ↑ Mood (inconclusive data).
7. Improve driving simulator steering performance.
8. Improve BP control (greater improvement seen in CPAP-adherent persons with more severe hypertension).
9. Improve heart function (LVEF) in persons with CHF.
10. ↓ Nocturia.
11. ↓ Healthcare utilization (physician claims and hospital stays).

Adverse consequences of PAP therapy for OSA
1. Aerophagia and gastric distention.
2. Arousals.
3. Barotrauma (e.g., pneumothorax, pneumomediastinum and pneumocephalus): Rare events.
4. Chest discomfort and tightness.
5. Claustrophobia.
6. Eye irritation (conjunctivitis).
7. Facial skin irritation, rash or abrasion.
8. Mask and mouth leaks.
9. Nasal congestion, dryness, epistaxis or rhinorrhea.
10. Noise from the device.
11. Sensation of suffocation or difficulty with exhalation.
12. Sinus discomfort or pain.

Adherence to PAP therapy
1. PAP use should be monitored objectively.
2. Objective compliance (use for > 4 hours per night for 70% of nights) ranges from 50-80%. Average nightly use: 5 hours.
3. Patterns of adherence to PAP therapy can often be discerned within the first few days of starting therapy.
4. Patients commonly overestimate their PAP utilization. *Really*.
5. PAP usage is not affected by the prescribed PAP level.
6. The following have *not* been demonstrated to consistently improve PAP compliance: (a) BPAP, (b) Cflex, (c) ramping mechanism, and (d) changing a problematic or poorly fitting nasal mask *after* therapy has been started.

Common reasons for non-adherence to PAP therapy
1. Difficulty with exhaling against high expiratory pressures: Consider Cflex or BPAP therapy.
2. Excessively high pressures: Consider trial of APAP, BPAP therapy, or adjunctive therapy with sleep position treatment or oral devices.
3. Gastric distention due to aerophagia: Consider BPAP therapy.

Effective approaches to improve PAP adherence
1. Patient education.
2. Heated humidification.

Factors predicting the need for heated humidification during PAP therapy
1. Age > 60 years.
2. Use of drying medications.
3. Presence of chronic nasal mucosal disease.
4. Prior UPPP.

Possible indications for BPAP therapy for OSA
1. Complaints of difficulty breathing out against high CPAP pressures.
2. Gastric distention due to aerophagia.
3. Concurrent obstructive or restrictive lung disease.
4. Concurrent hypoventilation syndrome with persistent O_2 desaturation despite CPAP therapy.

Possible indications for APAP for OSA
1. APAP titration: To identify a single fixed pressure for subsequent treatment with a conventional CPAP device. APAP devices are not recommended for split-night PAP titration. Non-snorers should not be titrated with APAP devices using diagnostic algorithms that rely solely on vibration or sound production.
2. APAP treatment: Used in a self-adjusting mode for nightly therapy of OSA.
3. Contraindications:
   a. CHF.
   b. Significant respiratory disease (e.g., COPD).
   c. Daytime hypoxemia and respiratory failure.
   d. Nocturnal O_2 desaturation unrelated to OSA (e.g., OHS).
4. Compared to conventional laboratory CPAP titration, APAP titration is associated with *no* significant differences in:
   a. Reductions in AHI and arousal indices.
   b. Changes in sleep architecture.
   c. SaO_2.
   d. Subsequent CPAP acceptance.
5. Compared to conventional CPAP, APAP is associated with:
   a. Lower mean airway pressure.
   b. Potentially higher peak airway pressure (in the presence of mouth or mask leaks).
   c. Similar objective compliance.
   d. Similar efficacy (elimination of respiratory events and improvement in EDS).

6. Published outcomes regarding one APAP model from a specific manufacturer may not necessarily be applicable to other systems.
7. Proper mask fitting is *crucial* prior to unattended APAP use.

Non-invasive positive pressure ventilation
1. May be considered for persistent sleep-related hypoventilation and CO_2 retention that persist despite PAP and supplemental O_2 therapy.

Oral devices for OSA
1. Indications:
   a. Snoring.
   b. Mild to moderate OSA.
   c. Severe OSA (in some).
2. Types:
   a. Mandibular repositioners: Displace the mandible and tongue anteriorly.
      i. The most commonly used oral devices.
   b. Tongue-retaining devices: Secure the tip of the tongue in a soft bulb located anterior to the teeth to hold the tongue in an anterior position.
      i. Preferred for edentulous persons or those with compromised dentition.
3. Benefits of oral devices for OSA:
   a. ↑ SaO_2.
   b. ↓ EDS.
   c. ↓ AHI.
   d. ↑ QOL.
   e. ↓ BP (less effective than PAP therapy).
4. Reported efficacy from 40-80%. Compliance is about 50-80%.
5. Contraindications:
   a. Inability to breathe nasally.
   b. Sleep apnea that is primarily central in nature.
   c. In growing children.
   d. Inadequate or compromised dentition (for mandibular repositioners).
   e. Significant TMJ dysfunction (for mandibular repositioners).
6. Complications:
   a. Dry mouth sensation.
   b. Excessive salivation.
   c. Dental pain.
   d. Undesirable dental movements (for mandibular repositioners).
   e. Jaw or TMJ pain.
7. Note:

   a. Follow-up PSG after optimal fit has been achieved is recommended to assure therapeutic efficacy as is periodic assessments by a dentist and sleep physician.

Summary:
1. *Mandibular repositioners for OSA: Chin out.*
2. *Tongue retainers for OSA: Tongue out.*

Upper airway surgery for OSA
1. General:
   a. Indicated primary for persons with definitive craniofacial or UA abnormalities responsible for OSA.
   b. PSG following UA surgery is recommended to determine its therapeutic efficacy. Long-term follow-up is required.
2. Types of surgery:
   a. *Tonsillectomy and adenoidectomy:*
      i. Particularly effective in childhood OSA due to adenotonsillar enlargement.
   b. *To increase dimensions of nasal airway:*
      i. Nasal surgeries: Septoplasty, polyp removal and turbinectomy.
   c. *To increase dimensions of retropalatal airspace:*
      i. Uvulopalatopharyngoplasty (UPPP): Excision of uvula, posterior portion of the soft palate, redundant pharyngeal tissue, and tonsils, and trimming of the tonsillar pillars. Note: Subsequent use of nasal CPAP may be compromised by UPPP with an increase in mouth leaks.
   d. *To increase dimensions of retrolingual airway:*
      i. Laser midline glossectomy and lingualplasty.
      ii. Tongue base reduction with hyoepiglottoplasty.
      iii. Genioglossal advancement.
      iv. Hyoid myotomy and suspension.
      v. Mandibular advancement.
   e. *To increase dimensions of retrolingual, retropalatal and transpalatal airway:*
      i. Uvulopalatopharyngoglossoplasty.
      ii. Maxillo-mandibular advancement.
   f. *To bypass upper airway:*
      i. Tracheotomy: Percutaneous tracheal opening. Indicated for severe life-threatening OSA that is

unresponsive to other types of therapy. The only surgical procedure that is consistently effective as a sole procedure for OSA.
3. Most effective surgical procedures for OSA:
   a. Tracheotomy.
   b. Bariatric surgery for weight management.
   c. Maxillo-mandibular advancement.

Summary:
What do you call a surgeon who performs the following procedures for OSA:
1. *Nasal septoplasty - Shape shifter.*
2. *Uvulopalatopharyngoplasty - Palate-thin-ian.*
3. *Lingualplasty - Tongue slasher.*
4. *Mandibular advancement - Jaw breaker.*
5. *Tracheotomy - Cut throat.*

Management of residual sleepiness despite PAP therapy
1. Assure optimal PAP pressure and adherence.
2. Distinguish EDS from fatigue.
3. Identify and manage other disorders that can give rise to EDS (e.g., insufficient sleep, narcolepsy or mood disorder).
4. Eliminate (if possible) use of sedating medications.
5. Modafinil or armodafinil may be considered as an adjunct therapy for improving alertness and wakefulness. Neither drug reverses the negative impact of OSA on cardiovascular morbidity. It should *not* be used to replace PAP therapy for OSA.

Upper airway resistance syndrome
1. Repetitive sleep-related episodes of decreased inspiratory airflow due to increasing UA resistance, and accompanied by increased or constant respiratory effort and arousals from sleep (i.e., RERAs).
2. Gender: M = F.
3. Consequences include sleep fragmentation, insomnia, EDS, and fatigue. May contribute to risk of systemic hypertension or hypotension. Other clinical features include headaches, myalgias, history of fainting, irritable bowel syndrome and PLMS.
4. Diagnostic caveats:
   a. UARS should be excluded in persons with unexplained EDS or presumptive idiopathic hypersomnia.
   b. Persons may have subtle physical examination findings such as cold extremities and postural hypotension during tilt table testing.
5. PSG features: $\uparrow$ WASO and $\downarrow$ N3. Alpha intrusion and bruxism may be present.
   a. AHI < 5. Respiratory events are not associated with O_2 desaturation. Snoring may be absent. Presence of EEG arousals following decrement in airflow and increased respiratory effort.
   b. Esophageal pressure monitoring (reference standard): Increasingly negative esophageal pressure [Pes] excursions preceding arousals, followed by less negative Pes excursions as airflow increases during arousals.
   c. Other diagnostic methods: Nasal pressure monitoring (inspiratory flattening followed by a rounded contour during arousals).
6. Therapy: PAP, oral devices or UA surgery.

Central Sleep Apnea

In this section
General
PSG features
Classification of CSA based on level of ventilation
Classification of CSA based on etiology
Primary central sleep apnea
Cheyne Stokes respiration
High altitude periodic breathing
Central sleep apnea due to medication use
Central sleep apnea due to congestive heart failure
Sleep-onset central apneas
Central sleep apnea during CPAP titration
Therapy of central sleep apnea

General
1. Repetitive cessation of airflow during sleep due to reduction or loss of ventilatory effort.
2. Can give rise to sleep fragmentation, insomnia or EDS. Persons with CSA may also be asymptomatic.
3. PSG is necessary for the diagnosis of CSA.

PSG features
1. Cessation of respiration and ventilatory effort lasting $\geq$ 10 seconds.
2. Respiratory events are most common during sleep onset and N1/N2 sleep.
3. RIP or strain gauge: Absence of chest and abdominal movement.
4. Diaphragmatic EMG: No respiratory muscle activity.
5. Esophageal pressure monitoring: No changes in pressure.
6. Nasal pressure monitoring: Rounded profile.
7. Oximetry: Generally milder O_2 desaturation than in OSA.
8. Snoring may occur but is less prominent than in OSA.
9. Diagnostic criteria:
   a. $\geq$ 5 central apneas per hour of sleep.

Classification of CSA based on level of ventilation
1. Hypercapnic:
   a. Hypoventilation during sleep (high sleep $PaCO_2$).
   b. Often associated with daytime hypoventilation (high waking $PaCO_2$).
   c. $\downarrow$ Ventilatory responsiveness to hypercapnia.
   d. Etiology:
      i. Central alveolar hypoventilation.
      ii. Neuromuscular disorders.
      iii. Chronic use of long-acting opioids.
2. Non-hypercapnic:
   a. Not associated with daytime hypoventilation (normal or low waking $PaCO_2$).
   b. $\uparrow$ Ventilatory response to hypercapnia.
   c. As $PaCO_2$ levels increase during sleep, brief arousals trigger a hyperventilatory "overshoot" that lowers $PaCO_2$ below its apneic threshold and gives rise to central apneas.
   d. Etiology:
      i. Idiopathic CSA.
      ii. Sleep-onset or post-arousal CSA.
      iii. CSA due to CHF.
      iv. High altitude periodic breathing.
      v. Complex sleep apnea.

Classification of CSA based on etiology
1. Primary (idiopathic).
2. Secondary to other medical disorders (more common than the primary form).
   a. Cardiac, renal and neurological (e.g., CHF, renal failure, brainstem lesions, head injury, neuromuscular disorders, stroke and autonomic dysfunction) disorders.
   b. Chronic use of long-acting opioids.

Primary central sleep apnea
1. Unknown etiology.
2. Rare condition. Gender: M > F. Prevalence greater in middle-aged and older adults.

Cheyne Stokes respiration
1. Periodic breathing with recurring episodes of crescendo-decrescendo ventilation separated by central apneas or hypopneas. Central apneas are post-hyperventilatory in

nature.

2. Present during NREM sleep, and improves or resolves during REM sleep.
3. Gender: M > F. Generally affects older adults > 60 years of age. Prevalence of 25-40% in CHF, and 10% in stroke. With CHF, risk factors include male gender, age > 60 years, atrial fibrillation and hypocapnia.
4. Pathophysiology:
   a. Prolonged lung-to-chemoreceptor circulation time (in some). Cycle length is related inversely to cardiac output and directly to circulation time.
   b. Lower daytime and sleep-related $PaCO_2$ levels (< 45 mm Hg).
   c. ↑ Hypercapnic respiratory drive.

High altitude periodic breathing
1. Cycles of central apnea and hyperpnea developing on ascent to high altitude (usually > 4,000-7,600 meters).
2. Risk factors include (a) greater hypoxic ventilatory drive, (b) higher elevation, (c) faster speed of ascent, and (d) male gender.
3. Occurs primarily during NREM sleep. Respiration becomes more regular during REM sleep.
4. Develops due to hypoxia-induced hyperventilation that results in hypocapnic alkalosis and central apneas. Mechanism: Hypoxia-induced hyperventilation ⇒ hypocapnic (low $PaCO_2$) alkalosis ⇒ CSA during sleep ⇒ $PaCO_2$ rises ⇒ resumption of ventilation ⇒ ventilatory overshoot ⇒ $PaCO_2$ falls below apneic threshold ⇒ CSA.
5. PSG features:
   a. ↑ WASO, ↑ N1, ↑ N2 and ↓ N3.
   b. Cyclic periods of central apneas and hyperpneas (cycle length of 12-34 seconds). Central apnea lasts ≥ 10 seconds, and is associated with O_2 desaturation.
   c. > 5 CAs per hour of sleep.

Central sleep apnea due to medication use
1. Depression of hypercapnic respiratory drive, with central apneas, periodic respiration, Biot breathing or hypoventilation, related to chronic use (≥ 2 months) of long-acting opioids (e.g., methadone).

Central sleep apnea due to congestive heart failure
1. CSA, CSR and OSA can develop in persons with CHF.
2. CSA is present in about 50% of persons with CHF. Prevalence and severity are correlated with LV function.
3. ↑ Mortality in CHF patients with CSR than in those without CSR.

Sleep-onset central apneas
1. Central apneas may develop if $PaCO_2$ (higher during sleep and lower during wakefulness) fluctuates above or below the apnea threshold.
2. Generally transient, and resolves as sleep progresses.
3. Repetitive sleep-onset central apneas can give rise to sleep-initiation insomnia.

Central sleep apnea during PAP titration
1. Also referred to as complex sleep apnea.
2. Development of CSA or CSR during acute application of CPAP in persons with predominantly obstructive or mixed apneas during the initial diagnostic study.
3. Estimated to occur in 15% of persons with OSA titrated with CPAP.

Therapy of central sleep apnea
1. Treatment of underlying causes (e.g., CHF).
2. Avoidance of respiratory depressants (e.g., BZ or opioid narcotics) in hypercapnic CSA.
3. O_2 therapy may benefit some persons with non-hypercapnic CSA (e.g., CSR). Indicated for high-altitude periodic breathing. May result in worsening hypercapnia in persons with hypercapnic CSA.
4. Inhaled CO_2 or addition of dead space (indications are not well established).
5. Pharmacologic therapy:
   a. Acetazolamide: For high-altitude periodic breathing.
   b. Theophylline: For CSA or CSR related to CHF, and for CSA related to immaturity in newborns.
   c. Medroxyprogesterone: For OHS.
   d. Hypnotic agents: For sleep-onset central apneas.
6. Positive airway pressure therapy:
   a. CPAP or BPAP for CSA or CSR due to CHF (might improve cardiac function but may have no benefit on mortality; monitor efficacy of therapy closely).
   b. ASV for complex sleep apnea.
7. Nocturnal non-invasive ventilation: For persons with hypercapnic CSA.

Hypoventilation Syndromes

In this section
General features
Medical and neurological disorders causing alveolar hypoventilation
Idiopathic alveolar hypoventilation
Congenital central alveolar hypoventilation syndrome

General features
1. Sleep-related O_2 desaturation.
2. Elevated $PaCO_2$ during sleep:
   a. $PaCO_2 > 45$ mm Hg, or
   b. $PaCO_2 < 45$ mm Hg but is abnormally increased relative to waking levels.
3. Waking ABG may be normal or abnormal.
4. Pathophysiology:
   a. ↓ Minute ventilation.
   b. ↓ TV.
   c. Abnormal V/Q relationships.
   d. Sleep-related reductions in ventilatory chemosensitivity and respiratory load responsiveness.
5. PSG features:
   a. ↑ SOL, ↓ SE, ↑ WASO, ↓ N3 and ↓ R.
   b. SaO_2 during sleep < 90% for > 5 minutes with a nadir ≥ 85%.
   c. > 30% of TST with $SaO_2 < 90\%$.
   d. ↑ $PaCO_2$.
6. Therapy:
   a. Treatment of underlying disorder/s.
   b. Ventilatory assistance during sleep.

Medical and neurological disorders causing alveolar hypoventilation
1. Respiratory disorders.
   a. Interstitial lung disease.
   b. Pulmonary hypertension.
   c. Lower airways obstruction (bronchiectasis or COPD): Risk of nocturnal hypoxemia is increased in (a) $FEV_1/FVC < 60\%$, (b) ↓ awake SaO_2, and (c) comorbid OSA [overlap syndrome].
   d. Chest wall disorders (kyphoscoliosis).
2. Neurological disorders.
   a. Amyotrophic lateral sclerosis.
   b. Diaphragm paralysis.
   c. Muscular dystrophy.
   d. Myasthenia gravis.
   e. Myopathy.
   f. Post polio syndrome.
   g. Spinal cord injury.
   h. Stroke (involving brainstem).

Idiopathic alveolar hypoventilation
1. No respiratory, chest wall or neuromuscular disorder. Normal respiratory mechanics.
2. Due to ↓ chemoresponsiveness to CO_2.
3. Hypoventilation is more pronounced during REM sleep.
4. Gender: M > F. Onset during adolescence or early adulthood.

Congenital central alveolar hypoventilation syndrome
1. Failure of automatic control of breathing.
   a. Hypoxemia and hypercapnia.
   b. ↓ Responsiveness of central and peripheral chemoreceptors to O_2 and CO_2.
2. Onset of hypoventilation usually in infancy. May present as respiratory failure, cyanosis, ALTE or cor pulmonale.
3. Hypoventilation is worse during sleep than wakefulness. More severe during N3 than REM sleep.
4. Associated features:
   a. Autonomic dysfunction (e.g., ↓ HR variability or ↓ BP).
   b. Hirschsprung's disease (in 16% of patients).
   c. Neural crest tumors (e.g., ganglioneuromas or ganglioneuroblastomas).
   d. Ocular abnormalities (e.g., strabismus).
   e. Swallowing dysfunction.
5. Rare condition. Gender: M = F.
6. Many cases involve de novo mutations of the PHOX2B gene. Autosomal dominant with incomplete penetrance.

Onset of Sleep Disorders across the Ages

In this section
Infancy
Childhood
Adolescence
Young adulthood
Mid- and older adulthood

Infancy
1. Benign sleep myoclonus of infancy.
2. Congenital central alveolar hypoventilation syndrome.
3. Primary sleep apnea of infancy.

Childhood
1. Confusional arousals.
2. Idiopathic insomnia.
3. Limit-setting sleep disorder.
4. Nightmare disorder.
5. Obstructive sleep apnea (pediatric).
6. Sleep enuresis.
7. Sleep-onset association disorder.
8. Sleep-related bruxism.
9. Sleep-related rhythmic movement disorder.
10. Sleep talking.
11. Sleep terrors.
12. Sleepwalking.

Adolescence
1. Behaviorally-induced insufficient sleep syndrome.
2. Delayed sleep phase disorder.
3. Idiopathic hypersomnia.
4. Inadequate sleep hygiene.
5. Narcolepsy.
6. Recurrent hypersomnia.
7. Recurrent isolated sleep paralysis.

8. Sleep-related hallucinations.
9. Sleep-related idiopathic non-obstructive alveolar hypoventilation.

Young adulthood
1. Catathrenia.
2. Excessive fragmentary myoclonus.
3. Idiopathic hypersomnia.
4. Narcolepsy.
5. Paradoxical insomnia.
6. Propriospinal myoclonus at sleep onset.
7. Psychophysiologic insomnia.
8. Restless legs syndrome.
9. Sleep-related eating disorder.
10. Snoring.

Mid- and older adulthood
1. Advanced sleep phase disorder.
2. Alternating leg muscle activation during sleep.
3. Cheyne Stokes breathing pattern.
4. Exploding head syndrome.
5. Familial fatal insomnia.
6. Hypnagogic foot tremor.
7. Obstructive sleep apnea (adult).
8. Periodic limb movement disorder.
9. Primary central sleep apnea.
10. REM sleep behavior disorder.
11. Sleep-related leg cramps.

The Early Years

In this section
General
Sleep architecture
Developmental milestones in sleep architecture
Sleep stages in the first 6 months of age
Sleep stages after 6 months of age
Developmental milestones in sleep patterns
Aggregate hours of sleep per day
Circadian rhythms and sleep homeostasis
Causes of insomnia in children
Nighttime waking
Behavioral treatment of childhood insomnia
Extinction techniques for childhood insomnia
Pharmacologic treatment of childhood insomnia
Excessive daytime sleepiness
Causes of sleepiness and fatigue in an adolescent or young adult (8Ds)
Childhood obstructive sleep apnea
Apnea of prematurity
Infant sleep apnea
Apparent life-threatening event
Snoring
Restless legs syndrome
Sleep in children with medical disorders

General
1. A child is not a small adult. There are significant differences in sleep architecture and manifestations of sleep disorders between children and adults.
2. Newborn sleep is polyphasic (i.e., occurring repetitively and randomly throughout the 24-hour day). Monophasic sleep (occurring once, generally at night) develops during early childhood (ages 3-5 years) when napping ceases.
3. Daily duration of sleep decreases from newborn infants (70% of 24-hour day) to adults (25-35% of 24-hour day).

Sleep architecture
1. In the 1st 6 months of life, sleep is classified as active sleep (REM sleep-equivalent), quiet sleep (NREM sleep equivalent), indeterminate sleep, or transitional sleep. Classification of sleep in infants older than 6 months of age is similar to that of adults (i.e., NREM or REM sleep).
2. Initial sleep episode can either be active [REM] sleep (< 3 months of age) or quiet [NREM] sleep (> 3-4 months of age).

3. Proportion of NREM-REM sleep is 50:50 in infants compared to 75:25 among adolescents and adults.
4. N3 sleep as percentage of TST is greatest during early childhood and declines with aging.
5. Percentage of REM sleep also decreases with aging, from 50% of TST (infants) to 25% of TST (adolescents and adults).
6. NREM-REM cycle length is ≈ 50-60 minutes during infancy and increases to ≈ 90-120 minutes in adults.
7. Neonates (newborn-2 months) are more likely to awaken from active rather than quiet sleep.

Developmental milestones in sleep architecture
1. Age at which specific sleep stages first appear:
   a. Active sleep: 28-30 weeks of gestation.
   b. Quiet sleep:
      i. Trace' discontineau: 32 weeks of gestation.
      ii. Trace' alternant: 36 weeks of gestation.

2. Age at which specific EEG features first develop:
   a. Sleep spindles: 1 month.
   b. Delta waves: 3 months.
   c. K complexes: 6 months.
   d. *Useful recall tool: 1-3-6 (SO-DO-KU).*
3. Development of distinct EEG features that allows differentiation among N1, N2 and N3 sleep occurs at 6 months.

Sleep stages in the first 6 months of age
1. Active sleep:
   a. First behavioral sleep state to appear. This is the predominant sleep state in the newborn period.
   b. Key features:
      i. Body and facial twitches and jerks.
      ii. Rapid eye movements.
      iii. Irregular respiration.
2. Quiet sleep:
   a. Becomes the predominant sleep state by 3 months of age.
   b. Key features:
      i. Minimal or no body movements.
      ii. Regular respiration.
   c. EEG patterns:
      i. High-voltage, slow-wave activity.
      ii. Trace' alternant (high voltage, slow activity interrupted by electrical silence) - present in the newborn and disappears by 1 month of age.
3. Intermediate sleep:
   a. Does not fully meet criteria for either active or quiet sleep.
4. Transitional sleep:
   a. Occurs in the transition between active, quiet and intermediate sleep.

Sleep stages after 6 months of age
1. Stage NREM 1:
   a. EEG: Desynchronized (low voltage, mixed frequency) activity.
   b. EOG: Absence of eye movements.
   c. EMG: Low muscle tone.
   d. Other features: Regular respiration and heart rate. Periodic breathing may be seen.
2. Stage NREM 2:
   a. EEG: Rhythmic activity (e.g., sleep spindles and K-complexes).
   b. EOG: Absence of eye movements.
   c. EMG: Low muscle tone.
   d. Other features: Regular respiration and heart rate.
3. Stage NREM 3:
   a. EEG: High voltage, slow (< 4 Hz) frequency activity.
   b. EOG: Absence of eye movements.
   c. EMG: Low muscle tone.
   d. Other features: Regular respiration and heart rate.
4. Stage REM:
   a. EEG: Desynchronized (low voltage, mixed frequency) activity.
   b. EOG: Episodic rapid eye movements (during phasic REM sleep).
   c. EMG: Muscle atonia.
   d. Other features: Irregular respiration and heart rate.

Developmental milestones in sleep patterns
1. There is great individual variability in the ages during which developmental milestones in sleep patterns occur. Therefore, a specific sleep behavior in a child may be considered "normal-for-age" or "problematic" depending on physiological maturity, cultural perceptions and parental expectations.
2. Greater frequency of awakenings among breast-fed compared to bottle-fed infants.
3. Age at which specific sleep-related behaviors commonly first develop:
   a. Longest sleep period occurring at night: 6 weeks.
   b. Nocturnal sleep consolidation (ability to sleep through the night): 6-9 months.
   c. Cessation of daytime napping: 3-5 years.

Aggregate hours of sleep per day
1. TST gradually decreases throughout childhood.
   a. Neonates (newborn-2 months): 16-19.
   b. Infants (2-12 months): 12-16.
   c. Toddlers (1-3 years): 11-12.
   d. Preschool (3-5 years): 10-12.
   e. Pre-adolescence (5-14 years): 8-11.
   f. Adolescence (14-18 years): 7-9.

   Note: Good rule to use:

< 2 months	*19*	
< 1 year	*15*	*(19 minus 4)*
1-3 years	*12*	*(15 minus 3)*
3-5 years	*10*	*(12 minus 2)*
> 5 years	*9*	*(10 minus 1)*

Circadian rhythms and sleep homeostasis
1. The SCN is functional *in utero*.
2. Irregular sleep-wake rhythms are present

immediately after birth. Regular sleep-wake rhythms develop by 2-4 months of age.
3. Endogenous circadian sleep phase preference (e.g., eveningness vs. morningness) first develops between 6-12 years of age.
4. Development of sleep phase delay between 12-18 years.
5. Marker for sleep homeostatic pressure is different for infants (theta activity [4-7 Hz]) compared to adults (delta activity [<4 Hz]).

Causes of insomnia in children
1. Adjustment sleep disorder (e.g. acute stress or change in bedroom environment).
2. Bedtime resistance: Generally starts with the development of autonomy and independence during the toddler years.
3. Colic: Sustained episodes of crying (> 3 hours), irritability or fussing, with no apparent reason. Onset generally at 3 weeks of age. Usually resolves by 3-4 months of age.
4. Food allergy.
5. Limit-setting sleep disorder: Repetitive refusal by a child to go to sleep at an appropriate time due to inadequate enforcement of bedtimes by the caregiver.
6. Nighttime fears (e.g., being left alone in the dark).
7. Psychophysiologic insomnia: Learned sleep-preventing associations and conditioned arousal.
8. Separation anxiety.
9. Sleep-onset association disorder: Inability to fall asleep, or return to sleep after an awakening, without the presence of certain desired, but inappropriate, objects or parental intervention.

Nighttime waking
1. Arousals normally occur every 90-120 minutes (i.e., 4-6 times each night).
2. ↑ Frequency of arousals with colic, parental co-sleeping and breastfeeding.
3. The infant's or child's ability to self soothe back to sleep without caregiver intervention determines whether spontaneous arousals are brief vs. prolonged and problematic.

Behavioral treatment of childhood insomnia
1. Parental education.
2. Maintenance of consistent bedtimes. Restful nighttime activities.

3. Age-appropriate bedtime.
4. Establishment of optimal bedroom environment.
5. Appropriate use of transitional objects (e.g., doll or blanket) for sleep-onset association disorder.
6. Consistent and predictable parental limit-setting for limit-setting sleep disorder.
7. Placing a child to bed while drowsy but still awake (to teach a child to fall asleep independently) beginning at 2-4 months of age.
8. Transitioning the infant to the final sleep environment (e.g., crib in infant's room) by 3 months of age.
9. Discontinuation of nighttime feedings in children ≥ 6 months of age.
10. Faded bedtime - Bedtime is progressively delayed (e.g., by 30 minutes) until the child is able to fall asleep rapidly. Subsequent bedtimes are then advanced or delayed depending on SOL until the desired bedtime is reached.
11. Positive bedtime routines – Establishing consistent and relaxing pre-bedtime activities.
12. Scheduled awakenings - The child is awakened by the parent slightly before the usual spontaneous time of awakening, reassured, and then allowed to return to sleep. Frequency of scheduled awakenings is progressively decreased until they are discontinued completely once the child is able to sleep through the night.
    a. Disadvantage is that children are not taught sleep initiation skills.
13. Extinction procedures.
14. Cognitive behavioral therapy: Sleep restriction, stimulus control and cognitive therapy as in adults.

Extinction techniques for childhood insomnia
1. Three general types, namely fast approach, gradual approach, or extinction with parental presence.
2. *Fast approach* (absolute extinction) involves putting the child in bed, leaving the child alone in the room, and ignoring inappropriate behavior and unreasonable demands until the next morning.
    a. Although generally effective within 3-7 days, a worsening of behavior ("extinction burst") may occur between 5-30 days from initiation of therapy.
3. *Gradual approach* (graduated extinction)

differs from the fast approach in that parents are allowed to respond to a child's inappropriate demands in a gradually decreasing fashion (i.e., longer duration between interventions or shorter period of intervention) until parental intervention is finally stopped.
4. *Extinction with parental presence* permits the parent to sleep in a separate bed in the child's bedroom but not to respond to any inappropriate behavior by the child.

Pharmacologic treatment of childhood insomnia
1. No hypnotic agent is currently approved by the US FDA for use in children. Neither the efficacy nor safety of melatonin has been established for children.

Excessive daytime sleepiness
1. EDS should be considered in any child > 5 years of age who (a) continue to nap during the day, especially if unplanned, or (b) sleep ≥ 2 hours more on weekends than on weekdays ("weekend oversleep").
2. Other common features:
   a. Falling asleep at inappropriate times and situations.
   b. Behavioral problems (inattentiveness, irritability, hyperactivity or impulsiveness).
   c. Cognitive problems or academic difficulties.
   d. Changes in mood (depression or anxiety).
   e. Fatigue and lethargy.

Causes of sleepiness and fatigue in an adolescent or young adult (8Ds)
1. Delayed sleep phase disorder (morning sleepiness).
2. Depression.
3. Deprivation (sleep).
4. Disorder (narcolepsy, idiopathic hypersomnia, hypothyroidism, recurrent hypersomnia, OSA or PLMD) .
5. Dope (illicit substance).
6. Drama (malingering).
7. Drinking.
8. Drugs (medications).

Childhood obstructive sleep apnea
1. Key features:
   a. EDS: Less common than in adults. Present in about 30% of children with OSA.
   b. Snoring.
   c. Witnessed apneas.
   d. Unusual sleep posture (e.g. hyperextended neck).
   e. Labored or paradoxical breathing. Thoracic retractions.
   f. Cognitive or behavioral difficulties.
2. Associated features:
   a. Sinus arrhythmia.
   b. Secondary enuresis.
   c. ALTE in infants.
   d. Bedtime resistance or problematic night waking.
3. Risk factors:
   a. Adenotonsillar enlargement. Most important risk factor in children. However, size of the tonsils and adenoids is not predictive of OSA in individual patients.
   b. + Family history.
   c. Excess body weight.
   d. Chronic nasal obstruction (e.g., allergies). Choanal atresia or stenosis.
   e. Craniofacial abnormalities (e.g., achondroplasia, Apert, Crouzon, Down, mucopolysaccharidoses, Pierre Robin and Treacher Collins).
   f. Prader-Willi syndrome.
   g. Cerebral palsy.
   h. Hypotonia and neuromuscular weakness.
   i. Arnold-Chiari malformation.
   j. Pharyngeal flap surgery to correct cleft palate.
4. Overall prevalence of 1-5% in children. Greatest prevalence between ages 2-6 years. May recur during adolescence in those successfully treated during childhood. Gender: M = F (in prepubertal children). Ethnicity: Higher prevalence in African-American and Asian than Caucasian children.
5. Consequences:
   a. Growth failure and developmental delay.
   b. Cognitive or behavioral problems (ADHD, aggressiveness, irritability or intellectual impairment).
   c. Mood disorder.
   d. Poor academic performance.
   e. Systemic and pulmonary hypertension.
   f. Nocturnal enuresis.
   g. Polycythemia.
   h. Chronic respiratory acidosis. Development of pectus excavatum.
   i. ↑ Frequency of parasomnias

(sleepwalking or sleep terrors).

6. Evaluation:
   a. History and physical examination.
   b. PSG. Consider monitoring end-tidal or transcutaneous CO_2.
   c. Radiologic studies (e.g., lateral cephalometric radiographs) for children with significant craniofacial abnormalities.
7. PSG features:
   a. Pauses in breathing or reduction in airflow by greater than 30-50% compared to baseline, lasting ≥ 2 normal respiratory cycles; ≥ 1 scoreable respiratory event per hour. Respiratory events are more common during REM sleep.
   b. Obstructive hypoventilation (prolonged periods of persistent partial UA obstruction with hypercapnia +/- O_2 desaturation).
   c. Sleep architecture is usually normal.
   d. Arousals (movement or autonomic) from sleep. May or may not be associated with EEG arousals.
   e. Paradoxical rib cage-abdominal wall motion.
   f. Sinus arrhythmia and other cardiac arrhythmias.
   g. O_2 desaturation and hypercapnia.
   h. Esophageal pressure monitoring: Markedly negative pressure swings.
   i. MSLT: Normal SOL.
8. Therapy:
   a. Adenotonsillectomy: Treatment of choice for most children with OSA. Assess therapeutic efficacy 6-8 weeks after surgery.
   b. Consider CPAP if UA surgery is not indicated, contraindicated or ineffective. Requires regular clinical and PSG reassessment.
   c. Oral devices may be tried in older adolescents when growth of craniofacial bones and UA soft tissues is largely complete.
   d. Nasal steroids for chronic nasal obstruction.

Apnea of prematurity

1. Obstructive or central apneas or hypopneas in infants < 37 weeks of gestation. Frequency: Mixed > central > obstructive apneas. May also present with periodic breathing.
2. Respiratory events may be associated with bradycardia, hypoxemia or need for caregiver intervention.
3. Prevalence is inversely related to gestational age at birth. Spontaneous resolution with maturation.

Infant sleep apnea

1. Obstructive or central apneas or hypopneas in infants > 37 weeks of gestation. Central events are more common than obstructive events. Respiratory events can be associated with hypoxemia, brady-tachycardia, cyanosis and arousals. They occur more frequently during REM sleep.
2. Risk factors include (a) low-birth weight, (b) medical and neurological disorders (anemia, lung disease, GER, metabolic derangements or infection), and (c) medication use, including anesthesia.
3. Infant sleep apnea is *not* an independent risk factor for sudden infant death syndrome (SIDS).
4. Decrease in apnea frequency after the early weeks of life.

Apparent life-threatening event

1. Clinical features include: (a) apnea, (b) change in color or tone (limpness), and (c) choking or gagging.

Snoring

1. All children should be screened for snoring.
2. Snoring in children may be associated with EDS, behavioral and cognitive problems (attention, language, memory and executive function), and mood disorders.
3. PSG is indicated to distinguish primary snoring from OSA.

Restless legs syndrome

1. Prevalence of 15% in children.

Sleep in children with medical disorders

1. Sleep disturbance in children can be due to:
   a. Allergies.
   b. Asthma.
   c. Atopic dermatitis.
   d. Colic.
   e. Congenital central alveolar hypoventilation syndrome.
   f. Cystic fibrosis.
   g. Gastroesophageal reflux.
   h. Irritable bowel syndrome.
   i. Otitis media.

2. Increased risk of OSA in children with:
   a. Achondroplasia.
   b. Cerebral palsy.
   c. Down syndrome.
   d. Juvenile rheumatoid arthritis.
   e. Meningomyelocele.
   f. Neuromuscular disorders.
   g. Prader-Willi syndrome.
   h. Sickle cell disease (due to adenotonsillar hypertrophy).

The Golden Years

In this section
General
Physiologic changes with aging
Sleep and sleep patterns
Sleep disorders
Changes in sleep architecture

General
1. Sleep requirements do not decline with aging.
2. Aging is associated with greater nocturnal sleep disturbance (prevalence of 50%), EDS and daytime napping.
3. While some of the sleep disturbance can be attributed to normal aging itself, most are due to comorbid medical (menopause or nocturia), neurological, psychiatric (depression), and primary sleep disorders, and the adverse effects on sleep of medications used to treat them.
4. Older women are better able to maintain satisfactory sleep with aging compared to older men.

Physiologic changes with aging
1. ↓ Melatonin secretion.
2. Earlier sleep onset and offset relative to melatonin secretion.
3. ↓ Amplitude of circadian sleep-wake rhythms.
4. Phase advancement of circadian sleep-wake rhythms and body temperature (in some).
5. ↓ Homeostatic sleep drive.
6. ↓ Arousal threshold (greater sensitivity to adverse environmental factors).
7. ↓ GH secretion during sleep.
8. ↑ Circadian nadir of cortisol level.

Sleep and sleep patterns
1. ↓ Sleep quality.
2. ↑ Sleep disturbance.
   a. ↑ Nighttime awakenings.
   b. Frequent daytime naps.
   c. Polyphasic sleep pattern (in some).
3. ↓ Tolerance to shift work and jet lag.
4. ↑ Tolerance to SD.

Sleep disorders
1. Greater prevalence of insomnia, OSA, CSA, RLS, PLMD, RBD and ASPD.
2. Insomnia.

   a. The most common sleep complaint among older adults. More frequently involves sleep-maintenance insomnia.
   b. Risk factors for insomnia with aging: Depression, disability, poor health, multiple medical disorders, respiratory symptoms, sedative use and widowhood.
   c. Rarely due exclusively to aging itself.
   d. Poorer correlation between subjective sleep complaints and objective PSG parameters in older women compared to older men.

Insomnia with aging: Men sleep less; women complain more.

3. Obstructive sleep apnea.
   a. More prevalent in men. Risk of OSA among women increases with menopause. HRT in menopausal women decreases the prevalence of OSA.
   b. Compared to younger adults:
      i. ↓ Frequency and ↓ severity of OSA-related EDS.
      ii. ↓ Risk of cardiopulmonary diseases.
      iii. AHI is less able to predict mortality risk.
      iv. ↓ Association with obesity, snoring and witnessed apneas.
      v. Similar PAP adherence rates.
4. Nocturia with aging may be due to ↓ urinary bladder capacity, ↓ urinary concentrating ability, prostatic enlargement (in men), detrussor overactivity, and OSA (weak correlation with AHI).

Changes in sleep architecture
1. ↓ SE, ↑ SOL, ↑ WASO, and ↓/= TST.
2. ↓ N3.
3. ↓ REM SL and ↓/= R.
4. ↑ Sleep stage shifts. ↓ NREM/REM cycles.
5. ↓ Sleep spindle and K complex density.
6. ↓ REM density.

Sleep in Women

In this section
Sleep and female hormones
Obstructive sleep apnea
Central sleep apnea
Insomnia with aging
Menstrual cycle
Dysmenorrhea
Endometriosis
Premenstrual syndrome
Premenstrual dysphoric disorder
Oral contraceptive use
Polycystic ovarian syndrome
Pregnancy
Pregnancy-induced hypertension (pre-eclampsia)
Labor and delivery
Postpartum period
Breast feeding
Co-sleeping with infant
Menopause and post-menopause
Aging
Hormone replacement therapy

General
1. Greater subjective complaints of insufficient or nonrestorative sleep as well as increased need for sleep compared to men.

Sleep and female hormones
1. Progesterone: ↑ EDS (due to UA congestion).
2. Estrogen: ↓ REM sleep.

Obstructive sleep apnea
1. OSA is less common in pre-menopausal women than in men.
   a. Risk of OSA increases in women during menopause.
   b. ↓ Prevalence of OSA among postmenopausal women who use HRT compared to women not on HRT.
   c. Note: Data do not conclusively support the use of HRT as therapy for OSA among postmenopausal women.
2. Pertinent physical characteristics in women that might decrease susceptibility to UA collapse during sleep (compared to men):
   a. Less neck soft tissue volume.
   b. Shorter pharyngeal airway length.
   c. Lower pharyngeal compliance during sleep.
3. Differences in clinical presentation (compared to men):
   a. ↓ Snoring.
   b. ↑ Insomnia.
   c. ↑ EDS and fatigue.
4. Differences in PSG features (compared to men):
   a. Lower AHI (when matched for body weight).
   b. Less supine position dependency of respiratory events.
   c. REM sleep-related respiratory events are more frequent during the follicular phase compared to the luteal phase in premenopausal women.
5. ↓ Survival rates compared to men with similar AHIs.

Central sleep apnea
1. Less common in premenopausal women than in men.
2. Lower hypopcapnic apneic threshold.

Menstrual cycle
1. Sleep quality can deteriorate prior to and during the first several days of menstruation.
2. Sleep-related complaints: Insomnia and EDS.
3. Causes of sleep disturbance: Abdominal bloating and cramping, anxiety, breast tenderness, headaches and mood changes.
4. Compared to the follicular phase, the luteal phase is associated with:
   a. ↑ Subjective sleepiness.

   b. ↑ SOL and ↓ SE.

   c. ↑ N2. ↑ Sleep spindles and ≈14 Hz frequency EEG power density.

   d. ↓ R.

5. Menstruation is associated with ↑ latency to N3.

Dysmenorrhea
1. Painful uterine cramps occurring during menses.
2. Sleep-related complaints: ↓ Sleep quality and EDS.
3. PSG features: ↓ SE.

Endometriosis
1. Presence of endometrial tissue outside the uterus (e.g., abdomen or pelvis).
2. Sleep-related complaints: Sleep disturbance secondary to pain.

Premenstrual syndrome
1. Abdominal bloating, greater irritability and increased fatigue occurring prior to menses. Symptoms remit with menses.
2. Sleep-related complaints: Insomnia, frequent awakenings, non-restorative sleep, unpleasant dreams or nightmares and EDS.
3. PSG feature: No significant changes in sleep architecture.

Premenstrual dysphoric disorder
1. Fatigue, mood changes and daytime impairment developing prior to menses.
2. Sleep-related complaints: Insomnia or EDS.
3. PSG features: ↓ SE, ↑ N2 and ↓ R.

Oral contraceptive use
1. ↑ Mean levels of melatonin.
2. ↑ Body temperature during sleep.
3. PSG features: ↑ N1, ↑N2, ↓/= N3 and ↓ REM SL.

Polycystic ovarian syndrome
1. Increased ovarian production of male sex hormones.
2. Irregular or absent menstrual cycles, infertility, weight gain, insulin resistance and hirsutism.
3. Increased risk for OSA. AHI appears to correlate with serum levels of testosterone.

Pregnancy
1. Changes in sleep quality:
   a. Worse during 1st trimester.
   b. Improves during 2nd trimester.
   c. Worst during 3rd trimester.
2. Common causes of sleep disturbance during pregnancy:
   a. Anxiety.
   b. Back pain.
   c. Breast tenderness.
   d. Dyspnea.
   e. Fetal movements.
   f. Heartburn and GER.
   g. Leg cramps.
   h. Nausea and vomiting (morning sickness).
   i. Nocturia.
   j. RLS.
   k. Snoring and OSA.
3. Increase in daytime napping.
4. PSG features:
   a. ↓ SE and ↑ WASO.
   b. ↑ TST (decreases by late pregnancy).
   c. ↑ N1, ↑ N2 and ↓/= N3.
   d. ↓ R (during late pregnancy).
5. Increase in risk for snoring, OSA, RLS/PLMD, nocturnal leg cramps and EDS.
   a. Significant OSA is relatively uncommon unless it was present prior to pregnancy.

Pregnancy-induced hypertension (pre-eclampsia)
1. Characterized by hypertension, proteinuria, pedal edema and headaches.
2. Higher prevalence of snoring, OSA and PLMS.
3. PSG features: ↑ WASO.

Labor and delivery
1. Compared to longer nighttime sleep duration (> 7 hrs), shorter TST (< 6 hrs) prior to labor and delivery is associated with longer labor and increased likelihood of cesarean delivery.

Postpartum period
1. Sleep-related complaints: EDS, cognitive impairment and changes in mood.
2. Increase in frequency of napping.
3. PSG features:
   a. ↓ SE, ↓ TST and ↑ WASO.
   b. ↓ N1 and ↓ N2.
   c. ↑ N3 (returning to baseline pre-pregnancy levels by 1-3 months postpartum).
   d. = R and REM SL.
4. Greater sleep disturbance in:
   a. First-time mothers (compared to multiparas).

b. Cesarean section delivery (compared to vaginal delivery).
5. Sleep-related conditions associated with postpartum depression: Insomnia. ↓ SE, ↓ TST and ↓ REM SL.

Breast feeding
1. PSG features (compared to bottle feeding):
   a. ↓/= TST, ↓ N1, ↓ N2 and ↑ N3.

Co-sleeping with infant
1. PSG features (compared to sleeping alone):
   a. ↑ WASO (but possibly shorter duration of individual arousals).

Menopause and post-menopause
1. Menopause is defined as the cessation of menstruation. Associated with declining estrogen and progesterone levels.
2. Common complaints include hot flashes, night sweats, insomnia, mood changes, fatigue and EDS.
3. Sleep-related conditions (compared to premenopause):
   a. ↑ Subjective complaints of sleep disturbance.

b. Increased prevalence of insomnia and OSA.
c. PSG features: ↑ SOL, ↓ SE, ↓ or ↑ TST, ↓ or ↑ WASO, ↑ N1, ↑ N3 and ↓ R.
4. Consider gabapentin for treatment of menopause-related hot flashes.

Aging
1. Sleep in healthy older women (compared to older men):
   a ↑ Frequency of insomnia.
   b. Poorer sleep quality.
   c. ↑ Need for daytime naps.
   d. ↑ Use of sedative-hypnotic agents.
   e. Less changes in sleep architecture (no significant ↓ in N3).

Hormone replacement therapy
1. Therapy with oral synthetic estrogens and progesterone.
2. Beneficial effects on sleep:
   a. Improvement in sleep quality.
   b. ↓ Prevalence of OSA, insomnia and hot flashes.
3. PSG effects of HRT: ↑ SE, ↓ SOL, ↑ TST, ↓ WASO and ↑ N3.

Gender

General
1. There are distinct gender differences in prevalence among many common sleep disorders.

Males > females
1. Catathrenia.
2. Cheyne Stokes breathing pattern.
3. High altitude periodic breathing.
4. Kleine Levin syndrome.
5. Limit-setting sleep disorder (uncertain).
6. Long sleeper.
7. Narcolepsy with cataplexy.
8. Obstructive sleep apnea (adults).
9. Primary central sleep apnea.
10. REM sleep behavior disorder.
11. Sleep enuresis (children).
12. Sleep-onset association disorder (uncertain).
13. Sleep-related coronary artery ischemia (due to OSA).
14. Sleep-related gastroesophageal reflux (with Barrett's esophagus).
15. Sleep-related idiopathic non-obstructive alveolar hypoventilation.
16. Sleepwalking (adults).
17. Sleep terrors (adults).
18. Snoring (adults).

Females > males
1. Adjustment insomnia.
2. Exploding head syndrome.
3. Fibromyalgia.
4. Insomnia due to mental disorder.
5. Nightmare disorder (adults).
6. Paradoxical insomnia (uncertain).
7. Psychophysiologic insomnia.
8. Restless legs syndrome.
9. Short sleeper.
10. Sleep enuresis (adults).
11. Sleep-related coronary artery ischemia (Prinzmetal angina).
12. Sleep-related dissociative disorder.
13. Sleep-related eating disorder.
14. Sleep-related hallucinations.

Males = females
1. Advanced sleep phase disorder.
2. Confusional arousals.
3. Congenital central alveolar hypoventilation syndrome.
4. Familial fatal insomnia.
5. Free-running circadian rhythm sleep disorder.
6. Idiopathic hypersomnia with long sleep time.
7. Nightmare disorder (children).
8. Obstructive sleep apnea (children, prepuberty).
9. Periodic limb movement disorder.
10. Recurrent isolated sleep paralysis.
11. Shift work sleep disorder.
12. Sleep-related bruxism.
13. Sleep-related epilepsy.
14. Sleep-related rhythmic movement disorder.
15. Sleep talking.
16. Sleep terrors (children).
17. Sleepwalking (children).

Two short rules
If you simply can't recall the preceding lists, remember these:

Males > females: SRBD
       RBD

Females > males: G*I*RLS
       N
       S
       O
       M
       I
       A

Legend:
1. *SRBD: Sleep-related breathing disorders (CSR, high altitude periodic breathing, OSA [adults] and CSA).*
2. *RBD: REM sleep behavior disorder.*
3. *Insomnia.*
4. *RLS: Restless legs syndrome.*

Polysomnography

Definitions

1. PSG involves the continuous and simultaneous recording of several physiologic variables during sleep (e.g., EEG, EOG, EMG, ECG, airflow, snoring, thoracic and abdominal movement, and SaO_2).
2. Other sensors that may be used during PSG include esophageal pressure monitors, $PetCO_2$, $PtcCO_2$, PAP level, additional EEG channels (for evaluation of suspected nocturnal seizures), video-monitoring (for evaluation of suspected parasomnias or seizures), and esophageal pH sensors (for evaluation of suspected GER).

Indications for PSG

1. Diagnosis of SRBD.
2. PAP titration for SRBD.
3. Follow-up after UA surgery or dental devices for OSA. (Note: Follow-up PSG is not routinely indicated for patients who have become, and remain, symptom-free while on effective CPAP therapy.)
4. Diagnosis of narcolepsy (followed by MSLT on the day following PSG).
5. Diagnosis of PLMD.
6. Evaluation of atypical or injurious parasomnias (with additional EEG derivations and video recording).
7. Evaluation of suspected nocturnal seizures (with additional EEG derivations and video recording).

Types of diagnostic sleep studies

1. Level 1: Attended in-laboratory full PSG. Gold standard for the diagnosis of OSA.
2. Level 2: Unattended full PSG (comprehensive portable PSG).
3. Level 3: Cardiorespiratory sleep studies, or

modified portable sleep apnea testing consisting of ≥ 4 bioparameters (e.g., airflow, SaO_2, respiratory effort, ECG or body position).

4. Level 4: Continuous 1 or 2 bioparameter recording (SaO_2 with or without airflow measurement).

The polygraph equipment

1. A polygraph, consisting of a series of AC and DC amplifiers and filters, records several physiologic variables during sleep.
2. High-frequency (fast) physiologic variables (e.g., EEG, EOG, EMG and ECG) are recorded using *AC amplifiers*.
   a. High-frequency filters are used to reduce fast, presumably non-physiologic, potentials.
   b. Low-frequency filters are used to reduce slow potentials that might interfere with proper recording.
   c. Note: If low filter settings are set too high, this can reduce the amplitude of delta waves and eye movements in the EEG and EOG, respectively.
3. Low-frequency (slow) physiologic variables (e.g., SaO_2 and CPAP levels) are recorded using *DC amplifiers*.
   a. DC amplifiers are not equipped with low-frequency filters.
4. Airflow and respiratory effort are recorded using either AC or DC amplifiers.
5. A derivation is the difference in voltage between 2 electrodes. It can be either bipolar or referential.
   a. *Bipolar*: Two standard electrodes are matched to each other.
   b. *Referential*: A standard electrode is matched to a reference electrode.

9 Basic steps in performing a PSG

1. A sleep diary is completed for 2 weeks before the study. PSG is performed during the patient's customary bedtime.
2. Questionnaires (including measures of sleepiness, such as ESS) are completed prior to the start of the study.
3. Placement of electrodes and sensors. Each channel is provided appropriate settings for sensitivity, and high- and low-frequency filters.
4. Biocalibrations are performed. Patients are asked to perform certain actions (e.g., look up and down, or breathe in and out) to check the integrity of the electrodes and amplifiers.

5. Study is started. Time when recording started ("lights out") is noted.
6. Monitoring and observation. Correction of artifacts, if present. Titration of PAP, if indicated.
7. Study is ended. The time the study ended is recorded ("lights on").
8. Biocalibrations are repeated.
9. Post-study questionnaires are completed.

Electroencephalography

1. Placement of EEG electrodes is based on the International 10-20 system. Each electrode is provided with a letter that represents the corresponding region of the brain and a numerical subscript.
2. Location of electrodes: frontal (F), central (C), occipital (O) and mastoid (M).
   a. Odd numbers are given for left-sided electrodes.
   b. Even numbers are used for right-sided electrodes.
   c. Z is used for for midline electrodes.
3. Recommended electrode placements are F4M1, C4M1 and O2M1. Backup electrode placements are F3M2, C3M2 and O1M2.
4. Alternative electrode placements are FzCz, CzOz and C4M1.
5. Additional EEG electrodes may be used when evaluating nocturnal seizure activity.

Basic EEG wave frequencies

1. The voltage recorded from EEG electrodes originates from the summed potential activity of cortical neurons.
2. Frequency of EEG waves [Hz]:
   a. Delta (< 4).
   b. Theta (4-7).
   c. Alpha (8-13).
   d. Beta (> 13).
3. *Useful mnemonic: Order of EEG waves based on increasing Hz:* **Do The AlphaBet** *or* **DTBA** *(delta, theta, beta, alpha).*
4. Delta waves:
   a. High-amplitude (peak to peak of > 75 μV).
5. Alpha waves:
   a. Amplitude is generally < 50 μV in adults.
   b. Present when a person is relaxed and drowsy and eyes are closed. Eye opening suppresses alpha activity.
   c. Most prominent in the occipital leads.
6. Beta waves:
   a. Present during alert wakefulness.

EEG waveforms

1. *K complex:*

a. High-amplitude, biphasic wave (an initial sharp negative deflection immediately followed by a positive high-voltage slow wave) with duration of ≥ 0.5 seconds.
b. Seen maximally over the vertex.

2. *Saw-tooth waves:*
   a. Theta waves with a notched waveform that occurs during REM sleep.
   b. More prominent over the vertex and frontal leads.

3. *Sleep spindles:*
   a. Brief oscillations with a frequency of 12-14 Hz lasting 0.5-1.5 seconds. Amplitude is generally < 50 μV.
   b. More prominent over the central leads. Generated in the midline thalamic nuclei.
   c. Seen in N2 and N3 sleep.
   d. "Pseudo-spindles" or "drug spindles" related to BZ use have a higher frequency (≈ 15 Hz).

4. *Vertex sharp deflections:*
   a. Sharp negative deflections with amplitude < 250 μV.
   b. Maximal over the vertex.

Electrooculography

1. Records the difference in potentials (dipole) between the cornea (positive) and the retina (negative).
   a. *Reminder: CO-PO (cornea = positive charge). RE-NE (retina = negative charge).*

2. This dipole changes with eye movements. A positive voltage (downward deflection) is recorded when the eye moves toward an electrode, and a negative voltage (upward deflection) accompanies an eye movement away from an electrode.
   a. *Reminder: PO-DO-TO (positive voltage = downward deflection = toward an electrode).*

3. Recommended electrode placements are E1M2 and E2M2.
   a. E1 = 1 cm below the left outer canthus.
   b. E2 = 1 cm above the right outer canthus.
   c. M2 = right mastoid process.

4. Alternative electrode placements are E1Fpz, E2Fpz.
   a. E1 = 1 cm below and 1 cm lateral to the left outer canthus.
   b. E2 = 1 cm below and 1 cm lateral to the right outer canthus.
   c. Fpz = midline frontoparietal.

5. May reduce electrode distance to 0.5 cm for children.

6. EOG electrodes are placed using adhesive and *not* collodion.

7. Conjugate eye movements create out-of-phase deflections in the two EOG channels. EEG artifacts produce in-phase deflections.

8. There are two general patterns of eye movements.
   a. *Slow rolling eye movements:* Occur during relaxed drowsiness with closed eyes, N1 sleep or brief awakenings.
   b. *Rapid eye movements:* Occur during waking with open eyes (eye blinks) or during REM sleep.

9. Use of SSRI or TCA may be associated with eye movements during N2 and N3 sleep (so called "Prozac eyes").

Electromyography (chin)

1. Location of three electrodes:
   a. Midline, 1 cm above the inferior edge of the mandible.
   b. 2 cm to the right of midline and 2 cm below the inferior edge of the mandible.
   c. 2 cm to the left of midline and 2 cm below the inferior edge of the mandible.
   d. May reduce electrode distance to 1 cm for children.

2. Derivation consists of either one of the electrodes below the mandible referred to the electrode placed above the mandible. The other inferior electrode can be used as a back-up if the initial electrodes fail.

3. An additional electrode may be placed over the masseter muscle to detect the presence of bruxism.

Electrocardiography

1. A single modified lead II with electrodes placed below the right clavicle near the sternum and over the lateral chest wall at the left 6th or 7th intercostal space.

2. Important cardiac rhythms:
   a. *Asystole:* Cardiac pause > 3 seconds in duration (for patients ≥ 6 years old).
   b. *Sinus bradycardia:* HR < 40 beats per minute (for patients ≥ 6 years old).
   c. *Sinus tachycardia:* HR > 90 beats per minute (for adult patients). Sinus rates are faster in young children.
   d. *Narrow-complex tachycardia:* HR > 100 beats per minute. At least 3 consecutive beats with QRS duration < 120 msec.
   e. *Wide-complex tachycardia:* HR > 100 beats per minute. At least 3 consecutive beats with QRS duration ≥ 120 msec.

f. *Atrial fibrillation*: Irregularly irregular rhythm with no consistent P waves.

Measuring airflow
1. Techniques include nasal pressure monitoring, pneumotachography, thermistors, thermocouples and $PetCO_2$ monitoring.
2. Pneumotachography is the reference standard for detecting obstructive apnea-hypopneas.
3. Thermal sensing devices and $PetCO_2$ monitoring provide indirect and qualitative measures of airflow.
4. With nasal pressure monitoring, obstructive respiratory events are associated with a plateau (flattening) of the inspiratory flow signal whereas central respiratory events are associated with reduced but rounded signals.
5. For identifying apneas, the recommended and alternative techniques are:
   a. Recommended: Oronasal thermal sensor.
   b. Alternative: Nasal air pressure transducer (adults). $PetCO_2$ or summed calibrated inductance plethysmography (children).
6. For identifying hypopneas, the recommended and alternative techniques are:
   a. Recommended: Nasal air pressure transducer.
   b. Alternative: Inductance plethysmography or oronasal thermal sensor.

Measuring respiratory effort
1. Techniques include esophageal pressure monitoring, surface diaphragmatic EMG, strain gauges, RIP or thoracic impedance.
2. Measurement of respiratory effort is important in distinguishing obstructive, central and mixed apneas.
3. Recommended sensor for measuring respiratory effort is esophageal manometry or inductance plethysmography.
4. Alternative sensor is diaphragmatic or intercostal EMG.

Measuring oxygenation and ventilation
1. Recommended sensor for O_2 saturation is pulse oximetry. Minimum acceptable signal averaging time is 3 seconds.

2. Recommended sensor for alveolar hypoventilation in children is $PtcCO_2$ or $PetCO_2$.

Pulse transit time
1. PTT refers to the transmission time for the arterial pulse pressure wave to travel from the aortic valve to the periphery (interval between the ECG R-wave and the subsequent pulse shock wave at the finger). It is typically about 250 msec.
2. PTT is inversely related to BP. PTT increases during inspiratory falls in BP, and decreases during arousal-induced increases in BP.
3. Persons with OSA have transient increases in BP accompanying arousals from sleep, and falls in BP during inspiration. PTT may be useful in distinguishing central and obstructive apnea-hypopneas.

Identifying snoring
1. Snoring can be detected using a microphone.

Electromyography (anterior tibialis)
1. Electrodes placed over the anterior tibialis of both legs are used to detect PLMS. Additional electrodes can be placed over the upper extremities (extensor digitorum communis) to identify RBD.

Technical specifications for electrodes and sensors
1. EEG and EOG:
   a. Desirable sampling rate (Hz)   500
   b. Minimal sampling rate (Hz)   200
   c. High frequency filter (Hz)   35
   d. Low frequency filter (Hz)   0.3
   e. Maximum impedance (K ohms) 5
2. EMG and snoring:
   a. Desirable sampling rate (Hz)   500
   b. Minimal sampling rate (Hz)   200
   c. High frequency filter (Hz)   100
   d. Low frequency filter (Hz)   10
3. ECG:
   a. Desirable sampling rate (Hz)   500
   b. Minimal sampling rate (Hz)   200
   c. High frequency filter (Hz)   70
   d. Low frequency filter (Hz)   0.3
4. Respiration:
   a. High frequency filter (Hz)   15
   b. Low frequency filter (Hz)   0.1
5. Oximetry:
   a. Desirable sampling rate (Hz)   25
   b. Minimal sampling rate (Hz)   10

6. Airflow, nasal pressure, esophageal pressure and chest/abdominal movements:
   a. Desirable sampling rate (Hz)   100
   b. Minimal sampling rate (Hz)   25

Scoring sleep stages: general considerations

1. PSG data are divided into 30-second time periods or epochs. The standard sleep study paper speed is 10 mm/second (30 cm per epoch page).
2. Identification of seizure activity is enhanced by faster paper speeds of ≥ 15 mm per second (preferably 30 mm per second), or adequate digital EEG sampling rates.
3. Each epoch is assigned a single sleep stage that comprises the greatest percentage of the epoch.

Scoring adult sleep stages

1. Stage W:
   a. > 50% of epoch has alpha EEG waves over the occipital region with eye closure.
   b. If alpha waves are absent, the presence of any of the following:
      i. Conjugate vertical eye blinks (0.5-2 Hz).
      ii. Reading eye movements (conjugate slow movement followed by a rapid movement in the opposite direction).
      iii. Voluntary rapid open eye movements.
   c. Usually relatively high chin EMG tone.
2. Stage N1:
   a. Alpha EEG waves are replaced by low voltage, mixed frequency (4-7 Hz) waves that occupy > 50% of the epoch.
   b. In persons who do not generate alpha waves, the start of:
      i. 4-7 Hz waves with slowing of background EEG activity by ≥ 1 Hz compared to stage W.
      ii. Vertex sharp waves with duration of < 0.5 seconds. Maximal over the central region.
      iii. Presence of slow eye movements. No rapid eye movements.
   c. Absence of K complexes and sleep spindles.
   d. Tonic chin EMG levels are typically lower than during relaxed wakefulness.
3. Stage N2:
   a. The start of stage N2 is defined by the presence of K complexes (not associated with arousals) or sleep spindles during the 1st half of the epoch or during the last half of the previous epoch if criteria for stage N3 are absent.
   b. The continuation of stage N2 is defined by the presence of low amplitude, mixed frequency EEG rhythms, and if the epoch contains, or is preceded, by K complexes (not associated with arousals) or sleep spindles.
4. Stage N3:
   a. ≥ 20% of the epoch is occupied by slow wave (0.5-2 Hz and > 75 μV) EEG activity over the frontal regions.
5. Stage R:
   a. Presence of all of the following:
      i. EEG: Low amplitude, mixed frequency activity.
      ii. EOG: Rapid eye movements.
      iii. Chin EMG: Low tone (lowest level in the study or at least no higher than the other sleep stages).
   b. The continuation of stage R is defined by the presence of low amplitude, mixed frequency EEG activity, low chin EMG tone, and no K complexes or sleep spindles in epochs that either contains rapid eye movements or that are preceded by stage R.
6. Major body movements:
   a. Presence of movement or muscle artifact that obscures the EEG for > 50% of the epoch.
      i. An epoch with a major body movement is scored the same stage as the epoch that follows it, but is scored as stage W if alpha rhythm is present or if it is preceded, or followed, by a stage W epoch.

Percentage of sleep stages in an adult

1. 50%-50% rule:
   a. 50% for N1 (5%) and N2 (45%).
   b. 50% for N3 (25%) and REM (25%).
2. The period from NREM stages 1-3 to REM sleep is called a sleep cycle. There are commonly 3-5 NREM-REM sleep cycles during the night, each occurring every 90-120 minutes in adults.
3. N3 sleep predominates in the 1st half of the night whereas REM sleep percentage is greatest during the 2nd half of the night.
4. Normal sleep in an adult is characterized by short sleep latency (< 15 minutes), high sleep efficiency (> 95%), and few and relatively brief awakenings. Sleep is typically entered into through NREM sleep.

Scoring pediatric sleep stages

1. These rules apply to infants ≥ 2 months post-term.
2. Stage W:
   a. > 50% of the epoch contains alpha or dominant posterior EEG rhythm.
3. Stage N1:
   a. Alpha or dominant posterior EEG rhythm is replaced by low amplitude, mixed frequency (4-7 Hz) waves occupying > 50% of the epoch.
   b. In those who do not generate a dominant posterior rhythm, the start of:
      i. 4-7 Hz waves with slowing of the background activity by ≥ 1-2 Hz compared to stage W.
      ii. Vertex sharp waves.
      iii. Slow eye movements.
      iv. Rhythmic anterior theta activity.
      v. Hypnagogic hypersynchrony.
      vi. Diffuse or occipital-predominant high amplitude 3-5 Hz rhythmic activity.
4. Stages N2, N3 and R:
   a. Same as adult scoring rules.
5. Stage N (NREM):
   a. If K complexes, sleep spindles and slow wave activity are absent in all epochs of NREM sleep.

Scoring sleep in newborn infants

1. Sleep scoring in newborns also follows an "epoch" approach using behavior, respiration, EEG, EOG and EMG data.
2. Sleep is classified as either active REM sleep or quiet sleep. The term "intermediate sleep" is used when epochs do not fully meet criteria for active or quiet sleep.
3. Stage wake:
   a. Behavior: Eyes open, visible movements and vocalizations.
   b. Respiration: Variable.
   c. EEG: Mixed slow wave (theta) pattern with occasional beta and delta waveforms.
   d. EOG: Waking eye movements.
   e. EMG: Sustained tone with bursts of phasic activity.
4. Stage active REM sleep:
   a. Behavior: Eyes closed, visible movements (facial grimaces, smiles or movements of body and limbs) and vocalizations.
   b. Respiration: Irregular.
   c. EEG: Low-voltage irregular pattern or mixed pattern.
   d. EOG: Positive.
   e. EMG: Low.
5. Stage quiet sleep:
   a. Behavior: Eyes closed and no body movements.
   b. Respiration: Regular.
   c. EEG: High-voltage slow pattern, trace alternant pattern or mixed pattern.
   d. EOG: Negative.
   e. EMG: High.
6. Definitions:
   a. *Respiration* is classified as either regular or irregular.
      i. Regular: Rate varies < 20 breaths per minute.
      ii. Irregular: Rate varies > 20 breaths per minute.
   b. *EEG* is classified as:
      i. High-voltage slow pattern: Continuous, medium- to high-amplitude (50-150 μV) waveforms. Frequencies from 0.5-4 Hz. Present during quiet sleep.
      ii. Low-voltage irregular pattern: Low-amplitude (14-35 μV) waveforms. Frequencies from 5-8 Hz. Present during active REM sleep.
      iii. Trace alternant pattern: Bursts of slow (0.5-3 Hz) high-amplitude waves, fast low-amplitude waves, and sharp waves (2-4 Hz) lasting several seconds interspersed with periods of relative quiescence (mixed frequency waveforms) lasting 4-8 seconds. Present during quiet sleep.
      iv. Mixed pattern: High- and low-voltage waveforms. Present during both quiet and active REM sleep.
   c. *EOG* is classified as either positive or negative.
      i. Positive - Rapid eye movements are present.
      ii. Negative - No rapid eye movements.
   d. *EMG* is classified as either high or low tonic activity.
      i. High: Tonic activity occupies > half of epoch.
      ii. Low: Tonic activity occupies < half of epoch.

Scoring arousals

1. Abrupt EEG frequency shift (e.g., alpha, theta or frequencies > 16 Hz but not spindles) lasting ≥ 3 seconds and preceded

by ≥ 10 seconds of stable NREM or REM sleep. In addition, REM sleep arousals must be accompanied by an increase in chin EMG that is ≥ 1 second in duration.

Summary:
1. *NREM arousals: Require changes in EEG.*
2. *REM arousals: Require changes in EEG and EMG.*

Scoring adult respiratory events
1. Apnea:
   a. Decrease in peak thermal sensor amplitude by ≥ 90% of baseline for a duration of ≥ 10 seconds.
   b. Events can either be obstructive, central or mixed.
      i. Obstructive: Inspiratory effort is present throughout the entire event.
      ii. Central: Inspiratory effort is absent throughout the entire event.
      iii. Mixed: Absent inspiratory effort in the initial part of the event followed by inspiratory effort.
2. Hypopnea:
   a. Decrease in nasal pressure by ≥ 30% of baseline for a duration of ≥ 10 seconds accompanied by ≥ 4% O_2 desaturation.
3. Respiratory effort-related arousal:
   a. Breaths associated with increasing respiratory efforts or flattening of the nasal pressure waveform with duration of ≥ 10 seconds. Event precedes an arousal. Does not meeting criteria for either apnea or hypopnea.
4. Hypoventilation:
   a. ≥ 10 mmHg increase in $PaCO_2$ during sleep compared to supine wake values.
5. Cheyne Stokes respiration:
   a. ≥ 3 consecutive cycles of crescendo-decrescendo amplitude in respiration *plus* either:
      i. Duration of CSR of ≥ 10 consecutive minutes, or
      ii. ≥ 5 central apneas/hypopneas per hour of sleep.

Scoring pediatric respiratory events
1. These rules apply to children < 18 yrs of age.
2. Apnea:
   a. ≥ 90% fall in signal amplitude lasting ≥ 2 missed breaths.
   b. Events can either be obstructive, central or mixed.

3. Hypopnea:
   a. ≥ 50% reduction in nasal pressure amplitude compared to baseline, associated with arousal, awakening, or ≥ 3% O_2 desaturation, lasting for a duration of ≥ 2 missed breaths.
4. Respiratory effort related arousal
   a. When using a nasal pressure sensor: Reduction in sensor signal to less than 50% of baseline levels, associated with flattening of the waveform, snoring, increase in $PtcCO_2$ or $PetCO_2$, or visible increase in work of breathing lasting ≥ 2 breath cycles.
   b. When using an esophageal pressure sensor: Progressive increase in inspiratory effort accompanied by snoring, increase in $PtcCO_2$ or $PetCO_2$, or visible increase in work of breathing lasting ≥ 2 breath cycles.
5. Hypoventilation:
   a. $PtcCO_2$ or $PetCO_2$ > 50 mmHg in > 25% of TST.
6. Periodic breathing:
   a. > 3 episodes of central apneas with duration of > 3 sec separated by ≤ 20 seconds of normal respiration.

Scoring movement events
1. Alternating leg muscle activation:
   a. ≥ 4 EMG bursts, 0.5-3 Hz in frequency, alternating between legs with duration of 100-500 msec.
2. Bruxism:
   a. Increase in chin EMG activity that is ≥ 2 time above the background EMG tone, separated by ≥ 3 seconds of stable EMG. Episodes are either brief or sustained.
      i. Brief episodes (0.25-2 seconds in duration occurring in a sequence of ≥ 3 episodes).
      ii. Sustained episodes (> 2 seconds in duration).
   b. ≥ 2 audible bruxism episodes per night.
3. Excessive fragmentary myoclonus:
   a. ≥ 5 EMG bursts (each with a usual maximum duration of 150 msec) per minute occurring for ≥ 20 min of NREM sleep.
4. Hypnagogic foot tremor:
   a. ≥ 4 EMG bursts, 0.3-4 Hz in frequency, with duration of 250-1000 msec.
5. Periodic limb movements of sleep:

a. $\geq$ 4 consecutive leg movements, each 0.5-10 seconds in duration with an amplitude $\geq$ 8 μV above resting EMG. Period lengths are 5-90 seconds between onsets of consecutive movements.

b. Leg movements on different legs are counted as 1 movement if they are separated by < 5 seconds between movement onsets

6. REM sleep behavior disorder:
   a. Either sustained chin EMG muscle activity, or excessive transient chin or limb EMG muscle activity, or both during REM sleep.

7. Rhythmic movement disorder:
   a. $\geq$ 4 individual movements, each with a frequency of 0.5-2 Hz and an amplitude $\geq$ 2 times above resting EMG tone.

Definitions of polysomnographic parameters

1. Apnea index (AI): Number of apneas per hour of sleep.
2. Apnea-hypopnea index (AHI): Number of apneas *plus* hypopneas per hour of sleep.
3. Alpha-delta: Alpha waves occurring during N3 sleep.
4. Arousal index: Number of arousals per hour of sleep.
5. Bedtime: Time when a person gets into bed and attempts to fall asleep.
6. Final awakening: Time when a person awakens for the final time.
7. Lights out (LO): Time when sleep recording started.
8. Lights on (LOn): Time when sleep recording ended.
9. Oxygen desaturation index (ODI): Number of O_2 desaturation events per hour of sleep.
10. Periodic limb movement index (PLMI): Number of periodic limb movements per hour of sleep.
11. REM sleep latency (REM SL): Time in minutes from the onset of sleep to the first epoch of REM sleep. [About 60-120 minutes in healthy adults].
12. Sleep efficiency (SE): Ratio of TST to TIB [(TST X 100)/TIB].
13. Sleep onset latency (SOL): Time from lights out to sleep onset (i.e., first epoch of any stage of sleep). [< 15-30 minutes in healthy adults].
14. Sleep onset REM period (SOREMP): Occurrence of REM sleep within 10-15 min of sleep onset.
15. Time in bed (TIB): Duration of monitoring between "lights out" to "lights on".
16. Total sleep time (TST): Sum of all sleep stages (NREM stages 1-3 sleep *plus* REM sleep) in minutes.
17. Wake time after sleep onset (WASO) - Time spent awake from sleep onset to final awakening.

Artifacts

1. Artifacts are unwanted recordings during PSG that arise either from faulty electrode placement, defective monitoring devices or amplifiers, or contamination by physiologic or environmental variables.
2. Artifacts can be generalized (affecting several or most channels) or localized (limited to a single channel).
   a. Generalized artifacts suggest a defective reference electrode that is common to the affected channels.
   b. Localized artifacts suggest a defect in the specific electrode itself.

5 Important PSG artifacts and troubleshooting strategies

1. 60 Hz interference:
   a. Dense, square-shaped EEG tracing.
   b. Due to (a) interference by 60 Hz electrical activity from power lines, (b) high and unequal electrode impedance, or (c) lead failure.
   c. Corrective measure/s:
      i. Fix electrode placement or change leads.
      ii. Use 60 Hz filter as a last resort.
2. Electrode popping:
   a. Sudden, sharp, high-amplitude deflections.
   b. Due to (a) pulling of electrode leads away from the skin by body movements or respiration, (b) patient lying on the electrode, (c) faulty electrode placement, or (d) drying out of the electrode gel.
   c. Corrective measure/s:
      i. Fix electrode placement or change lead.
      ii. Apply more electrode gel.
3. EMG artifact:
   a. Discharges due to high EMG tone.
   b. Corrective measure/s:
      i. Fix electrode placement or change lead.
4. Prosthetic eye ("glass eye" artifact):
   a. No movement in the enucleated eye.

5. Sweat artifact:
    a. Slow undulating movements that are synchronous with respiration.
    b. Due to alterations in electrode potentials by salt in sweat.
    c. Corrective measure/s:
        i. Decrease room temperature.

Knowing the Tests

In this section
Epworth sleepiness scale
Stanford sleepiness scale
Multiple sleep latency test
Maintenance of wakefulness test
Actigraphy

Epworth sleepiness scale

1. Eight-item questionnaire that measures a person's general propensity to fall asleep in various situations in recent times:
   a. Sitting and reading.
   b. Watching television.
   c. Sitting and inactive in a public place.
   d. As a passenger in a car for an hour without a break.
   e. Lying down to rest in the afternoon.
   f. Sitting and talking to someone.
   g. Sitting quietly after lunch without drinking alcohol.
   h. Stopped in a car for a few minutes in traffic.
2. Chances of dozing: 0 (never), 1 (slight chance), 2 (moderate chance) or 3 (high chance).
3. Aggregate score: 0-9 (normal), $\geq$ 10 (sleepiness present; sleep specialist advice recommended).
4. Key points:
   a. Correlation between ESS, MSLT and MWT is poor.
   b. $\uparrow$ ESS score in persons with OSA. Score improves with effective therapy of OSA.

Stanford sleepiness scale

1. Seven-point subjective measure of perception of sleepiness at a given time, ranging from "wide awake, vital and alert" to "unable to remain awake with sleep onset imminent".

Multiple sleep latency test

1. An objective measure of the physiologic tendency to fall asleep in quiet situations.
2. Indicated for evaluation of unexplained EDS, or suspected narcolepsy, and to distinguish between narcolepsy and idiopathic hypersomnia.
3. Technical considerations:
   a. Adequate sleep duration and regular sleep-wake schedules should be maintained for $\geq$ 1-2 weeks prior to MSLT.
   b. Medications that can affect SOL and REM sleep (e.g., stimulants, hypnotics, sedatives, REM suppressants and opioids) should be discontinued for $\geq$ 2 weeks (or $\geq$ 5 times the half-life of the drug and its longest-acting metabolite) before the study.
   c. A nocturnal PSG should be performed immediately before an MSLT to exclude other causes of EDS (e.g., OSA or PLMD). An MSLT should not be performed after a split-night PSG.
   d. There should be an adequate duration of nocturnal sleep ($\geq$ 6 hours) during the preceding PSG.
   e. OSA, if present, should be adequately treated before performing an MSLT.
   f. If the patient uses PAP for OSA, it should be used during PSG and MSLT.
   g. The study consists of 4-5 nap opportunities. Each nap trial is 20 minutes in duration, performed every 2 hours starting about 1.5-3 hours after awakening from the previous night's sleep.
   h. Smoking and stimulating activities should be stopped before each nap trial. Caffeine and vigorous physical activity should be avoided during the day of the study.
   i. A urine drug screen should be performed during test day.
   j. Standard biocalibrations are performed before and after each trial.
   k. During the trial, the patient is asked to lie down in a comfortable position in a dark, quiet room, close his/her eyes and *try to fall asleep.*
   l. Standard leads include EEG, EOG, chin EMG and ECG.
   m. SOL is defined as the time from lights out to the onset of sleep (i.e., 1st epoch of any stage of sleep for clinical MSLT). If no sleep occurs during a nap trial, its

SOL is recorded as 20 minutes. In addition, the occurrence of SOREMPs (> 15 seconds of REM sleep in a 30-second epoch) is determined for each nap trial. REM SL is the time from the 1st epoch of sleep to the beginning of the 1st epoch of REM sleep.

n. The nap trial is terminated after 20 minutes if no sleep is recorded. If sleep is recorded, the test is continued for an additional 15 minutes to allow REM sleep to occur. The test is stopped after the 1st epoch of unequivocal REM sleep.

o. The patient is asked to get out of bed and to remain awake between nap trials.

p. A shorter 4-nap test may be considered if ≥ 2 SOREMPs have already occurred during earlier nap trials, and if the mean SOL is abnormal.

4. Test highlights:
   a. SOL tends to be shortest during the 3rd (noon) and 4th (early afternoon) naps and longest in the 5th nap (late afternoon).
   b. Short mean SOL suggests the presence of EDS.
      i. Mean sleep latencies (mean +/-SD [minutes]):
         1. Normal controls, 4-nap MSLT: 10 +/- 4
         2. Normal controls, 5-nap MSLT: 11 +/- 5
         3. Narcolepsy: 3 +/- 3
         4. Idiopathic hypersomnia: 6 +/- 3
      ii. A short SOL is present in up to 15-30% of normal individuals. Other causes of a short SOL include SD, DSPD, OSA, PLMD, acute withdrawal of stimulant agents, and use of long-acting hypnotic agents on the night preceding MSLT.
      iii. Normative MLST parameters are not well established for children < 8 years of age.
   c. Propensity for REM sleep is greatest during the 1st nap.
      i. Causes of SOREMPs include narcolepsy, OSA, DSPD, withdrawal from REM suppressants, alcohol withdrawal, depression and SD. SOREMPs is present in 1-3% of normal healthy adults.

Maintenance of wakefulness test
1. An objective measure of a person's ability to remain awake in quiet situations for a specified period of time.
2. Indicated to assess an individual's ability to maintain wakefulness, and to assess response to treatment for EDS.
3. Technical considerations:
   a. Consists of 4 nap opportunities performed at 2-hour intervals. A *40-minute* protocol for each nap is recommended. The 1st nap trial is started about 1.5-3 hrs after the person's customary wake time.
   b. The need for a PSG prior to MWT should be individualized as determined by the clinician.
   c. During each nap trial, a person is asked to sit in bed in a semi-reclined position and in a dark, quiet room. The person is instructed to *try to stay awake* during the test. However, measures to stay awake (e.g., singing) are not allowed during nap trials.
   d. Use of tobacco, caffeine and stimulant agents should be avoided during test day. Drug screening may be considered.
   e. Standard biocalibrations are performed before and after each nap trial.
   f. Standard leads include EEG, EOG and chin EMG.
   g. The nap trial is terminated if:
      i. Unequivocal sleep occurs (i.e., 3 consecutive epochs of N1 sleep, or 1 epoch of any other sleep stage); or
      ii. No sleep is recorded after 40 minutes.
4. SOL is defined as the time from lights out to the first epoch of sleep (sleep onset) for each nap. SOL correlates with the ability to stay awake.
   a. Mean SOL < 8 minutes is considered abnormal.
   b. Mean SOL > 8 minutes but < 40 minutes is of uncertain significance.
   c. Mean SOL = 40 minutes is considered normal. This may provide an appropriate expectation for individuals who require the highest level of alertness for safety.
5. Factoid: The MWT is less sensitive than MSLT in measuring sleepiness.

Actigraphy

1. A technique to determine periods of inactivity (rest or sleep) or activity using sensors that can detect movement.
2. Movements are detected using accelerometers that are typically worn on the wrist. Data can be recorded over a period of several days to weeks.
3. Movement data are summated for a specified epoch time, and each epoch is scored as either "active" or inactive" based on predetermined thresholds for activity counts.
4. Data that can be obtained with actigraphy include total wake time, TST, SOL (if used with an event monitor to mark the time when a person desires to fall asleep) and WASO.
5. Actigraphy is indicated for the evaluation of certain circadian rhythm sleep disorders and their response to therapy. It may also be considered to aid in the diagnosis of insomnia, particularly paradoxical insomnia.
6. Actigraphy monitoring should include ≥ 3 consecutive 24-hour periods.
7. Three most important features of actigraphy.
   a. It is better at measuring TST than identifying SOL.
   b. Degree of correlation between PSG and actigraphy for TST, total awake time, and sleep continuity is greater among normal sleepers than in persons with insomnia or sleep disturbances.
   c. PSG tends to detect more sleep time compared to actigraphy in both normal sleepers and in persons with insomnia.

Sleep Architectural Designs

In this section
General patterns of sleep architecture
High sleep input architecture pattern
Low sleep input architecture pattern
Circadian rhythm sleep patterns
Other factors affecting sleep architecture
Factors affecting REM sleep

General patterns of sleep architecture
1. There are 3 general patterns of PSG features, namely:
   a. High sleep input pattern: ↓ SOL, ↑ SE, ↑ TST and ↓ WASO.
   b. Low sleep input pattern: ↑ SOL, ↓ SE, ↓ TST and ↑ WASO.
   c. Circadian rhythm sleep patterns: Variable sleep architecture depending on whether PSG is performed during the conventional or habitual sleep schedule.
2. High sleep input pattern is associated with:
   a. Sleep deprivation.
   b. Disorders presenting with EDS.
   c. Sedating medications.
3. Low sleep input pattern is associated with:
   a. Disorders presenting with insomnia.
   b. Stimulant medications.

Sleep disorders with *high* sleep input architecture pattern
1. Narcolepsy.
   a. However, ↓ SE, ↓ TST and ↑ WASO in some persons.
2. Recurrent hypersomnia.
   a. However, ↓ SE and ↑ WASO.
3. Idiopathic hypersomnia.
   a. TST may be normal in Idiopathic hypersomnia *without long sleep time* type.
4. Behaviorally-induced insufficient sleep syndrome.

Sleep disorders with *low* sleep input architecture pattern
1. Insomnia.
   a. Adjustment insomnia.
   b. Psychophysiologic insomnia: Sleep architecture may be normal (reverse first-night effect with better sleep than usual during the 1st sleep laboratory night).
   c. Idiopathic insomnia.
   d. Inadequate sleep hygiene.
   e. Exceptions to rule:
      i. Paradoxical insomnia: Normal SOL and TST > 6.5 hours despite subjective reports of little or no sleep.
      ii. Limit-setting sleep disorder: Normal sleep architecture.
      iii. Sleep-onset association insomnia: ↑ SOL and ↑ WASO in the absence of desired circumstances. Normal TST and sleep quality when the required associations are met.
2. OSA. ↓ SOL (in some).
3. Restless legs syndrome.
4. Periodic limb movement disorder. ↓ SOL (in some if not accompanied by RLS).
5. Environmental sleep disorder (when PSG is performed in the person's home).
   a. PSG performed in the sleep laboratory: Normal sleep architecture.
6. Medical, neurological or psychiatric disorders:
   a. Asthma.
   b. COPD.
   c. Restrictive lung disease.
   d. Fibromyalgia.
   e. Sleep-related GER.
   f. Dementia.
   g. Sleep-related epilepsy.
   h. Sleep-related headaches.
   i. Major depression.
   j. Manic disorder.
   k. Anxiety disorder.
   l. Schizophrenia (acute psychotic decompensation).
   m. Personality disorder (obsessive-compulsive disorder).

Circadian rhythm sleep patterns
1. Delayed sleep phase disorder.
   a. When PSG is performed during conventional sleep schedule: ↑ SOL and ↓ TST.

b. When PSG is performed during habitual sleep schedule: Normal sleep architecture.
2. Advanced sleep phase disorder.
   a. When PSG is performed during conventional sleep schedule: ↓ or normal SOL, ↓ TST, and early wake time.
   b. When PSG is performed during habitual sleep schedule: Normal sleep architecture.
3. Irregular sleep-wake rhythm.
   a. 24-hour PSG performed over several days: Variable and disorganized pattern of sleep and wake.
4. Free-running disorder.
   a. PSG recorded at a fixed time period daily over several days: Progressively ↑ SOL and ↓ TST.
   b. Normal SE.
5. Jet lag.
   a. ↓ SE and ↑ WASO.
   b. Eastward travel: ↑ SOL (with habitual bedtime at destination).
   c. Westward travel: ↓ SOL (with habitual bedtime at destination).

6. Shift work sleep disorder.
   a. ↓ SE and ↑ WASO.

Other factors affecting sleep architecture
1. Aging: ↓ N3.
2. Recovery from SD: ↑ N3 and ↑ R.
3. Antidepressant use: ↑ REM SL and ↓ R.
4. "First-night effect" (sleeping in unfamiliar situations): ↓ N3 and ↓ R.

Factors affecting REM sleep
1. ↑ REM SL.
   a. Advance in bedtime or first-night effect.
   b. Alcohol (use).
2. ↓ REM SL.
   a. Alcohol (withdrawal).
   b. Delay in bedtime, including DSPD.
   c. Depression.
   d. Narcolepsy (SOREMPs).
   e. Normal healthy adults (in 1-3%).
   f. OSA (secondary to SD).
   g. SD (especially REM sleep deprivation).
   h. Schizophrenia.
   i. Sudden withdrawal of REM-suppressing agents.

Pharmacopeia Mnemonica

In this section
General
Antidepressants
Hypnotic agents
Stimulants
Antipsychotics
Opioids
Drugs of abuse
Common medications and substances that can cause insomnia
Common medications and substances that can cause sedation
Common medications that can cause or worsen RLS or PLMD
Common medications that can cause or worsen RBD
Common medications that can cause or worsen abnormal dreams or nightmares
Common medications affecting NREM sleep
Common medications affecting REM sleep

General
1. Medications can be sedating ($\downarrow$ SOL, $\uparrow$ SE, $\downarrow$ WASO and $\uparrow$ TST [high sleep input pattern]) or alerting ($\uparrow$ SOL, $\downarrow$ SE, $\downarrow$ TST and $\uparrow$ WASO [low sleep input pattern]), or both, as a direct action, adverse reaction or withdrawal effect.

Antidepressants
1. $\uparrow$ N3, $\uparrow$ REM SL and $\downarrow$ R.
2. Sudden discontinuation can cause REM sleep rebound. MAOIs are the most potent REM inhibitors.
   a. Exceptions to this rule:
      i. Increase in REM sleep: Bupropion and nefazodone.
      ii. No change in REM sleep: Mirtazapine and trimipramine.
      iii. Inconsistent effect on REM sleep: Trazodone.
      iv. Decrease or no change in N3 (in some): SSRI, MAOI.
3. SSRIs can cause abnormal slow eye movements during NREM sleep (so called "Prozac eyes").
4. SSRIs can be both sedating or alerting. Fluvoxamine and paroxetine are among the most sedating. Citalopram and fluoxetine are alerting.
5. Trazodone can cause postural hypotension and priapism.
6. Protriptyline increases UA muscle tone.
7. TCAs are associated with anti-cholinergic adverse effects (blurred vision, constipation, dry mouth, orthostatic hypotension, tachycardia and urinary retention.
   a. Sedating TCAs: Amitriptyline, doxepin and imipramine.
   b. Alerting TCAs: Protriptyline.
8. Antidepressants can induce or worsen RLS or PLMD. Exception to this rule: Bupropion.
9. SSRIs can induce RBD.

Hypnotic agents
1. Barbiturates, BZ receptor agonists and chloral hydrate act via the GABA receptor complex. They are sedating (high sleep input pattern).
2. BZ receptor agonists also decrease N3 and REM sleep. REM sleep rebound (with nightmares) may develop during drug withdrawal.
   a. Exception to this rule: Eszopiclone, zaleplon and zolpidem have minimal effect on N3 and REM sleep.
3. Rebound insomnia following BZ discontinuation is more severe with short-acting compared to longer-acting agents.
4. BZ can increase both spindle (12-14 Hz) and "pseudo-spindles" (14-18 Hz) density.
5. Barbiturates and BZ can worsen snoring and OSA.

Stimulants
1. Alerting (low sleep input pattern). Also $\downarrow$ N3 and $\downarrow$ R.
2. Withdrawal can give rise to EDS ($\downarrow$ SOL and $\uparrow$ TST) and $\uparrow$ R (REM sleep rebound).
3. Mechanisms of action:
   a. Increase in the synaptic availability of the monoamine transmitters, dopamine, serotonin and norepinephrine

(amphetamine, cocaine and
methylphenidate).
   b. Adenosine receptor antagonist and
inhibition of phosphodiesterase
(caffeine).
   c. Increase in cortical cholinergic
neurotransmission (nicotine).
   d. Alteration of hypocretin, dopamine,
GABA and histamine neurotransmission
(modafinil).
4. Modafinil is indicated for EDS secondary to
narcolepsy and SWSD. It is also used for
residual sleepiness in persons with OSA
who are being treated with PAP therapy.
5. Pemoline, a dopamine agonist stimulant,
has been withdrawn from the market due to
concerns regarding fatal liver failure.

Antipsychotics
1. Generally sedating (high sleep input pattern)
and ↓ R.
   a. Most sedating: Chlorpromazine,
clozapine, olanzapine, quetiapine and
thioridazine.
2. Changes in sleep architecture:
   a. ↑ REM SL: Chlorpromazine, haloperidol,
olanzapine and thiothixene.
   b. No change in REM SL: Risperidone and
quetiapine.
   c. ↑ N3: Olanzapine, risperidone and
thioridazine.
   d. No change in N3: Quetiapine and thiothixene.
   e. ↓ N3: Clozapine.

Opioids
1. Generally sedating (high sleep input
pattern).
2. PSG features during opioid use include ↓
N3 and ↓ R.
3. Insomnia and nightmares can develop
during opioid discontinuation.
4. They may worsen OSA, but improve
symptoms of RLS.

Drugs of abuse
1. Cocaine:
   a. Use: ↓ TST and ↓ R.
   b. Withdrawal (acute): ↑ TST and ↑ R.
2. Heroin: ↓ TST, ↓ N3 and ↓ R.
3. Marijuana (tetrahydrocannabinol [THC]):
   a. Low doses (sedating): ↑ TST, ↑ N3 and
slight ↓ R.
   b. High doses (hallucinatory): ↓ N3 and ↓
R.

   c. Withdrawal: ↑ SOL, ↓ TST and ↑ R
(rebound).

Common medications and substances that can cause insomnia
1. Alcohol (withdrawal from).
2. Anorectic agents.
3. Antidepressants.
   a. Bupropion.
   b. Fluoxetine.
   c. Protriptyline.
   d. Venlafaxine.
4. Antihypertensives.
   a. Metoprolol.
   b. Propanolol.
5. Antiparkinsonian drugs.
   a. Levodopa (high doses).
6. Bronchodilators.
   a. Albuterol.
   b. Theophylline.
7. Decongestants.
   a. Phenylpropanolamine.
   b. Pseudoephedrine.
8. Nicotine.
9. Steroids.
   a. Prednisone.
10. Stimulants.
   a. Caffeine.
   b. Cocaine.
   c. Dextroamphetamine.
   d. Methamphetamine.
   e. Methylphenidate.
   f. Modafinil.

Common medications and substances that can cause sedation
1. Anticonvulsants.
   a. Carbamazepine.
   b. Gabapentin.
   c. Phenobarbital.
   d. Phenytoin.
   e. Tiagabine.
   f. Valproic acid.
2. Antidepressants.
   a. Amitriptyline.
   b. Desipramine.
   c. Doxepin.
   d. Fluvoxamine.
   e. Imipramine.
   f. Lithium.
   g. Mirtazapine.
   h. Nefazodone.
   i. Nortriptyline.
   j. Paroxetine.
   k. Trazodone.
3. Antiemetics.

a. Metoclopramide.
b. Ondansetron.
c. Phenothiazines.
d. Scopolamine.
4. Antihistamines (first generation H1 agents).
a. Diphenhydramine (tolerance develops rapidly).
5. Antiparkinsonian drugs.
a. Pramipexole.
b. Ropinirole.
6. Antipsychotics.
a. Chlorpromazine.
b. Clozapine.
c. Haloperidol.
d. Olanzapine.
e. Thioridazine.
7. Barbiturates.
8. Benzodiazepine receptor agonists.
9. Chloral hydrate.
10. Gamma-hydroxybutyrate (sodium oxybate).
11. Melatonin and melatonin receptor agonists (ramelteon).
12. Muscle relaxants.
13. Narcotic agents.
14. Neuroleptic agents.

Common medications that can cause or worsen RLS or PLMD
1. Antidepressants (MAOI, SSRI and TCA).
2. Lithium.

Common medications that can cause or worsen RBD
1. Alcohol (withdrawal).
2. Antidepressants (MAOI, SSRI, TCA and venlafaxine).
3. Barbiturates.
4. Caffeine.

Common medications that can cause or worsen abnormal dreams or nightmares
1. Alcohol (withdrawal).
2. Amphetamines.
3. Antidepressants (MAOI, SSRI and TCA).
4. Antipsychotics.
5. Barbiturates.
6. Benzodiazepines.
7. Beta-blockers (propranolol).

8. Corticosteroids.
9. Donepezil.
10. Levodopa.
11. Mirtazapine.
12. Naproxen.
13. Opioids.
14. Reserpine.

Common medications affecting NREM sleep
1. Increase N3 sleep.
a. Alcohol (acute ingestion).
b. Carbamazepine.
c. Gabapentin.
d. Gamma hydroxybutyrate.
e. Lithium.
f. Mirtazapine.
g. Nefazodone.
h. Trazodone.
2. Decrease N3 sleep.
a. Alcohol (withdrawal).
b. Barbiturates.
c. Benzodiazepines.
d. Stimulants.

Common medications affecting REM sleep
1. Increase REM SL.
a. Antidepressants (MAOI, SSRI, TCA and venlafaxine).
b. Stimulant agents (amphetamine).
2. Decrease REM SL.
a. Bupropion.
b. Withdrawal of REM-suppressing agents.
3. Increase REM sleep.
a. Alcohol (withdrawal).
b. Bupropion.
c. Nefazodone.
d. Reserpine.
e. Withdrawal of REM-suppressants.
4. Decrease REM sleep.
a. Alcohol (acute ingestion).
b. Antidepressants (MAOI, SSRI, TCA and venlafaxine).
c. Stimulants (amphetamines and methylphenidate).
d. Barbiturates.
e. Benzodiazepines.
f. Lithium.
g. Narcotic agents.

Alcohol

In this section
General
Associated sleep disturbances
PSG features
PSG predictors of ethanol relapse during abstinence
Alcohol-dependent sleep disorder

General
1. Effects on sleep neurotransmitters: Facilitates GABA and inhibits glutamate.
2. Alcohol has a biphasic effect on sleep and waking.
   a. Stimulating: At low doses and on the rising phase of alcohol levels. *Note: Visualize an animated person having fun at a bar.*
   b. Sedating: At high doses and on the falling phase of alcohol levels. *Note: Visualize a drowsy person driving home after leaving the bar.*

Associated sleep disturbances
1. Alcohol use:
   a. ↑ Nightmares and vivid dreams.
   b. ↑ Enuresis.
   c. ↑ Restless legs.
   d. ↑ Sleep terrors and sleepwalking.
   e. ↑ Snoring and worsen OSA.
2. Acute alcohol withdrawal:
   a. Insomnia.
   b. Frequent awakenings accompanied by headaches and diaphoresis.
   c. Vivid, disturbing dreams.
3. Alcohol abstinence:
   a. Sleep disturbance, including insomnia, can persist for several years.
   b. ↓ TST with delirium tremens.

PSG features
1. Acute alcohol ingestion:
   a. ↓ SOL, ↓ WASO, ↑ N3, ↑ REM SL and ↓ R (first part of sleep period).
   b. ↑ WASO, ↓ N3 and ↑ R (second part of sleep period).
2. Alcohol withdrawal:
   a. ↑ SOL, ↑ WASO, ↓ TST, ↓ N3, ↓ REM SL and ↑ R (REM rebound).
3. Alcohol abstinence
   a. ↓ TST, ↑ WASO and ↓ N3.

PSG predictors of ethanol relapse during abstinence
1. ↓ N3, ↓ REM SL and ↑ R.

Alcohol-dependent sleep disorder
1. Habitual use of alcohol prior to anticipated bedtime only for its sedative effects. No other patterns of behavior compatible with overt alcoholism are present.

Genes and Sleep

General
1. Many physiologic processes and clinical disorders related to sleep are, at least in part, under genetic control.

Sleep architecture
1. Higher degree of concordance in MZ than DZ twins for TST, SOL, arousals, percentages of sleep stages, and density of rapid eye movements.

Circadian rhythms
1. Circadian rhythms are controlled by autoregulated transcription-translation positive and negative feedback loops involving clock-related proteins and other regulatory factors.
2. Mammalian circadian genes consist of *B-mal1, Casein kinase 1 (CK1), Clock (clk), Cryptochrome (Cry1* and *Cry2), Period (per1, per2* and *per3),* and *Timeless (tim).* Other genes may be involved.
3. An individual's chronotype ("eveningness" or "morningness") may be determined, in part, by the *Clock* gene.

Advanced sleep phase disorder (familial)
1. Autosomal dominant variant of the disorder with a serine to glycine mutation in the casein kinase I epsilon (CKIε) binding region of *hPer2 (human Period* 2) that is localized near the telomere of chromosome 2q. This causes hypophosphorylation of the hPer2 protein by CKIε and results in shortening of the transcription-translation feedback loop cycle duration.

2. Mutation in the gene coding for casein kinase I delta has also been reported.

Delayed sleep phase disorder
1. A positive family history may be present in 40% of affected persons.
2. An autosomal dominant pattern of transmission has been described in a family with DSPD.
3. Polymorphisms in the circadian clock genes, *hPer3, Clock, CKIε,* and *arylalkylamine N-acetyltransferase,* have been reported.

Insomnia
1. Higher concordance in MZ than DZ twins for insomnia symptoms.
2. Mutation in the gene coding for a GABA-A β3 subunit has been described.

Fatal familial insomnia
1. Autosomal dominant disease involving a single point mutation at codon 178 of the prion protein gene on chromosome 20.
2. Severity of the disease is influenced by codon 129, which can either be methionine homozygous (more severe and shorter duration of illness before death) or methionine-valine heterozygous (milder disease).

Narcolepsy
1. Risk of developing narcolepsy is 10-40 times greater among 1st degree relatives than in the general population.
2. Low concordance (25-30%) among MZ twins (suggesting environmental trigger factors).
3. Associated with certain human leukocyte

antigens (HLA).
 a. DR2 (particularly the subtype DR15).
 b. DQ1 (particular DQ6 [DQB1*0602]).
 c. DQB1*0602: The most important allele. Present in 90% of narcolepsy with cataplexy and 40-60% of narcolepsy without cataplexy. Most multiplex family cases (multiple members of the family having narcolepsy) are HLA DQB1*0602 positive. However, it is neither sensitive nor specific for narcolepsy (it is also prevalent in the general population and most persons positive for HLA DQB1*0602 do *not* have narcolepsy).
4. ↓ CSF hypocretin levels.
 a. Canine model: Mutation of hypocretin receptor-2 gene (Hcrt2) transmitted in an autosomal recessive fashion.
 b. Rodent model: Knockout mice for the precursor ligand for the hypocretin receptor.
 c. Human research: Pre-pro-hypocretin gene mutation in a case of early onset narcolepsy.

Idiopathic hypersomnia
1. Some persons may have an autosomal dominant mode of transmission.
2. Association with HLA-Cw2 in some familial cases.

Obstructive sleep apnea
1. ↑ Prevalence in 1st degree relatives.
2. Risk and severity of OSA is associated with apolipoprotein ε4 gene.
3. Hypertension in OSA is associated with polymorphism in the angiotensin-converting enzyme (ACE) gene.
4. Cardiovascular disease is associated with polymorphism in haptoglobin genotype.

Snoring
1. Higher degree of concordance in MZ than DZ twins.

Congenital central alveolar hypoventilation syndrome
1. Many cases involve *de novo* mutations in the PHOX2B gene. Autosomal dominant with incomplete penetrance.

Parasomnias
1. Higher degree of concordance in MZ than DZ twins for sleepwalking, sleep terrors, sleep enuresis and idiopathic sleep paralysis.
2. RBD: Association with HLA-DQB1*05 and DQB1*06 in some.
3. Sleepwalking: Association with HLA DQB1*0501.
4. Sleep bruxism: Up to 50% of persons may have a positive family history.
5. Sleep enuresis:
 a. Increasing prevalence related to the number of affected parents.
  i. 80% when both parents were enuretic as children.
  ii. 40% when one parent has a history of enuresis.
 b. Linkage to genes on chromosomes 12q, 13q and 22q has been described.

Restless legs syndrome
1. Positive family history in 90% of persons with primary RLS and 10% of persons with secondary RLS.
2. Autosomal dominant transmission with incomplete penetrance in up to 30-60% of primary RLS.
3. Higher degree of concordance in MZ than DZ twins.
4. Presence of 3 susceptibility loci (chromosomes 9p, 12q and 14q).

Medical Disorders

In this section
Allergic disorders
Cardiovascular disorders
Gastrointestinal disorders
Infectious disorders
Intensive care unit syndrome
Renal disorders
Respiratory disorders
Rheumatologic disorders
Miscellaneous disorders

Allergic disorders
1. Allergies.
   a. Sleep-related complaints: Insomnia.
   b. Allergic rhinitis can increase UA resistance and exacerbate OSA.
2. Atopic dermatitis.
   a. Sleep-related complaints: Sleep disturbance (due to frequent scratching), insomnia or EDS.
   b. PSG features: Low sleep input pattern.

Cardiovascular disorders
1. Hypertension.
   a. OSA is a risk factor for HTN independent of known confounding factors. Odds of hypertension increase by 1% for each additional apneic event per hour of sleep, and by 13% for each 10% decrease in nocturnal SaO_2.
   b. Loss of nocturnal fall in BP ("dipping" phenomenon) in OSA.
   c. Improvement in BP during PAP therapy in persons with co-existing OSA and hypertension.
2. Coronary artery disease.
   a. Risk of CAD is increased in middle-aged persons with OSA. Possible mechanisms include:
      i. Endothelial dysfunction.
      ii. Hypercoagulability: ↑ Plasma fibrinogen levels, ↑ platelet activity and ↓ fibrinolytic capacity.
      iii. Insulin resistance.
      iv. ↑ Pro-inflammatory cytokines (e.g., TNF-α, IL-6 and IL-8) and adhesion molecules (ICAM-1 and VCAM-1).
      v. Oxidative stress.
      vi. ↑ Sympathetic activity during sleep.
3. Congestive heart failure.
   a. ↑ Prevalence of OSA, CSA and CSR in persons with CHF. CSR occurs predominantly during N1 and N2 sleep.
   b. ↑ Levels of norepinephrine in CHF persons with CSA compared to those without CSA.
   c. OSA may contribute to worsening LV dysfunction.
   d. ↑ Mortality in CHF persons with (a) worse AHI and (b) increased left atrial size.
4. Cardiac arrhythmias.
   a. ↓ Prevalence of PVCs during sleep (due to greater parasympathetic tone).
   b. ↑ Prevalence of ventricular arrhythmias during arousals from sleep.
   c. In OSA, HR slows at the onset of the apneic episode and increases after the termination of the event.

Gastrointestinal disorders
1. Gastroesophageal reflux.
   a. Backflow of gastric acid and other gastric contents into the esophagus due to incompetent barriers at the gastroesophageal junction (i.e., transient relaxation of the lower esophageal sphincter and, to a lesser extent, upper esophageal sphincter). Episodes occur more frequently during wake compared to sleep, when GER develops during brief arousals.
   b. Sleep-related GER is associated with longer acid contact time (due to delayed esophageal acid clearance and decreased production of neutralizing saliva during sleep).
   c. Sleep-related complaints: Sleep fragmentation, insomnia, EDS, nocturnal heartburn, dyspnea, coughing, choking, retrosternal chest pain, or a bitter or sour taste.
   d. Prevalence of nighttime symptoms in patients with GER is about 80%.

Prevalence increases with aging and, perhaps, OSA.

 e. Chronic course. Complications include morning hoarseness, esophagitis, esophageal strictures, Barrett esophagus, chronic cough, asthma exacerbation, pharyngitis, laryngitis, bronchitis, pneumonia, and pulmonary fibrosis.

 f. Diagnosis requires continuous esophageal pH testing during PSG (arousals may accompany episodic reductions in distal esophageal pH).

  i. Abnormal esophageal manometry may be present (decreased lower esophageal sphincter pressure, more frequent transient lower esophageal sphincter relaxations, and diminished amplitude of peristalsis).

 g. PSG features: Repeated arousals followed by swallowing (i.e., increase in chin EMG activity). ↓ N3.

 h. Treatment: Elevation of head of bed. Histamine-2 antagonists or proton pump inhibitors. Anti-reflux surgery.

 i. Useful factoid:

  i. PAP therapy decreases frequency of nocturnal GER in patients with or *without* OSA!

2. Peptic ulcer disease.

 a. Patients with PUD have greater gastric acid secretion during sleep compared to normal healthy individuals.

 b. Sleep-related complaints: Repeated arousals and awakenings, and nocturnal abdominal pain (onset is commonly within the 1st 4 hours of sleep).

3. Functional bowel disorders.

 a. Chronic gastrointestinal symptoms are not associated with significant anatomical, metabolic or infectious abnormalities and include functional dyspepsia and irritable bowel syndrome.

 b. Sleep-related complaints: Poor sleep quality, frequent awakenings, nighttime abdominal discomfort and non-restorative sleep.

 c. PSG parameters are generally normal.

Infectious disorders

1. Sleeping sickness.

 a. Human African trypanosomiasis caused by *Trypanosoma brucei* or *Trypanosoma rhodesiense*. Transmitted by the bite of an infected tsetse fly.

 b. Two stages of human disease, namely an initial hemolymphatic stage (fever, cervical adenopathy and cardiac arrhythmias) and a terminal meningo-encephalitic stage (excessive sleepiness, sensory deficits and abnormal reflexes). Culminates in altered consciousness, cachexia, coma and eventually death, if untreated.

 c. Sleep-related complaints: EDS, insomnia (not uncommon) and reversal of sleep-wake periods.

 d. Endemic in certain regions of intertropical Africa.

 e. PSG features: Few vertex sharp waves, sleep spindles and K complexes. ↓ REM SL (SOREMPs).

 f. Diagnosis: Demonstration of pathogen in the blood, bone marrow, lymph node aspirates or CSF.

 g. Therapy: Anti-parasitic medications.

2. Human immunodeficiency virus (HIV) infection.

 a. About 1/3 of patients develop sleep disturbance.

 b. Sleep-related complaints: Insomnia, sleep fragmentation and EDS.

 c. PSG features: ↓ SOL, ↓ SE, ↑ WASO, ↓ N2 and ↑ N3 (↓ N3 in terminal stages).

 d. Antiviral therapy for HIV infection can disturb sleep. Efavirenz use can give rise to insomnia, frequent awakenings and vivid dreams.

3. Infectious mononucleosis.

 a. Sleep-related complaint: EDS.

4. Lyme disease.

 a. Multisystem (rheumatologic, neurological and dermatologic) disease caused by *Borrelia burghdorferi*. Human disease is transmitted via tick bites.

 b. Sleep-related complaints: EDS, insomnia, frequent awakenings, RLS and nocturnal leg jerking.

  i. Sleep disturbances can persist for several years.

 c. PSG features:

  i. ↑ SOL, ↓ SE and ↑ WASO.

  ii. Alpha waves may intrude into NREM sleep.

  iii. MSLT: Normal SOL.

Intensive care unit syndrome

1. Reversible mental status changes (e.g., delirium, disorientation or hallucinations) that develop 3-7 days after ICU admission, and

resolve within 48 hours of ICU discharge. Most important etiologic factor is SD.
2. Sleep-related conditions: Insomnia, EDS and reversal of sleep-wake patterns.
3. Sleep disturbance can be due to factors related to the patient (pain, anxiety or acute illness), diagnostic or therapeutic interventions (medication administration or routine nursing care), or to the ICU environment (noise or constant lighting).
4. PSG features: Low sleep input pattern.
5. Important factoids:
   a. Nurse observations of sleep time often overestimate objective measures of sleep duration.

Renal disorders
1. End-stage renal disease.
   a. Sleep disturbance can develop in about 60% to 80% of patients with ESRD.
   b. Sleep-related complaints: EDS, insomnia or reversal of day-night sleep patterns.
      i. High prevalence of OSA, RLS and PLMD.
   c. PSG features:
      i. ↑ SOL, ↓ SE, ↑ WASO and ↓ TST (low sleep pressure pattern).
      ii. ↑ N1, ↑ N2 and ↓ N3.
      iii. ↓ R.

Respiratory disorders
1. Asthma.
   a. Episodic dyspnea, wheezing or coughing due to reversible broncho-constriction and airway hyperreactivity to specific and nonspecific stimuli.
   b. Sleep-related complaints: Insomnia, sleep fragmentation, EDS and nocturnal hypoxemia.
   c. Possible mechanisms responsible for nocturnal bronchoconstriction include circadian variability in airflow (lowest in the early morning) and sleep-related changes in autonomic nervous system activity (greater parasympathetic tone and decrease in sympathetic activity), lung capacity, and inflammatory mediators. Episodes may be precipitated or aggravated by GER.
   d. Diagnosis is aided by ↓ in evening peak expiratory flow rates or ↓ FEV_1 compared to daytime values.
   e. PSG features: Low sleep input pattern.

   f. Therapy consists of combined inhaled corticosteroid and long-acting bronchodilator (e.g., salmeterol). Short-acting beta-agonists (e.g., albuterol) for acute control of asthma symptoms. PAP therapy for patients with concurrent asthma and OSA.
2. Chronic obstructive pulmonary disease.
   a. Progressive, not fully reversible, airflow limitation. Includes emphysema and chronic bronchitis.
   b. Sleep-related complaints: Repetitive awakenings, insomnia, non-restorative sleep or EDS. Nocturnal hypoxemia and hypercapnia in advanced disease.
   c. Factors responsible for sleep disturbance include nocturnal coughing or dyspnea, hypoxemia and hypercapnia, and medications (e.g., methylxanthines and beta-adrenergic agonists).
   d. Nocturnal O_2 desaturation may develop in moderate to severe disease. Episodes of O_2 desaturation are more frequent, of greater duration, and more severe during REM sleep compared to NREM sleep.
   e. The occurrence and severity of O_2 desaturation during sleep are influenced by baseline lung function, and awake PaO_2 and $PaCO_2$ (significant O_2 desaturation is more likely with lower PaO_2 or SaO_2, and higher $PaCO_2$).
   f. Mechanisms responsible for sleep-related O_2 desaturation: (1) hypoventilation (most important), (2) ventilation-perfusion (V/Q) mismatching, and (3) decrease in lung volumes.
   g. Sleep-related hypoxemic episodes appear to be more common among persons with chronic bronchitis than in those with emphysema. Persons with chronic bronchitis generally have lower baseline SaO_2, larger falls in SaO_2, more episodes of O_2 desaturation, and longer duration of O_2 desaturation during sleep than persons with emphysema.
   h. PSG features: Low sleep input pattern.
   i. Useful information: Frequency of arousals in COPD is *not* related to the degree of nighttime hypoxemia.
   j. "Overlap syndrome" refers to the presence of both COPD and OSA. Compared to isolated COPD, overlap syndrome is associated with lower

PaO_2, higher $PaCO_2$ and higher mean pulmonary artery pressures. PAP therapy is indicated for overlap syndrome.

   k. Therapy consists of long-acting beta-agonists (e.g., salmeterol) or long-acting anticholinergic agents (e.g., tiotropium). O_2 therapy may be considered for significant nocturnal O_2 desaturation. There is no evidence that treating nocturnal O_2 desaturation alone, in the absence of daytime hypoxemia, improves survival.

3. Cystic fibrosis.
   a. Autosomal recessive multisystemic disease. Abnormal sodium and chloride transport across the epithelium results in bronchiectasis, exocrine pancreatic insufficiency, intestinal and urogenital dysfunction, and abnormal sweat gland function.
   b. Sleep-related conditions: Sleep fragmentation, nocturnal coughing and sleep-related hypoxemia.

4. Diaphragm paralysis.
   a. Sleep-related conditions: Nocturnal hypoxemia (worse during REM sleep) and SRBD.

5. Restrictive pulmonary diseases.
   a. Reduced lung volumes due to disorders involving the lung parenchyma, pleura or chest wall. Include kyphoscoliosis, interstitial lung disease and severe obesity.
   b. Sleep-related conditions: Sleep disturbance, frequent awakenings, non-restorative sleep, EDS, SRBD (OSA and CSA), and nocturnal O_2 desaturation (transient or sustained).
   c. Hypoxemia is worse during REM sleep compared to NREM sleep.
   d. Remember: Deterioration of lung function may occur with CPAP therapy in persons with kyphoscoliosis.
   e. PSG features: Low sleep input pattern.

6. Obesity.
   a. Sleep-related complaints: Snoring, OSA, OHS and nocturnal hypoventilation.
   b. PSG features: Normal SOL, ↓ SE, normal REM SL and ↓ R.

Rheumatologic disorders

1. Fibromyalgia.
   a. Multiple tender areas throughout the body and fatigue.
   b. Sleep-related complaints: Nonrestorative sleep. Severity of daytime symptoms may decrease with improved sleep quality.
   c. Prevalence of 2% in the general population. Gender: F (80% of cases) > M.
   d. PSG: Low sleep input pattern and ↓ N3. Alpha EEG activity may be present during NREM sleep.
   e. Key points:
      i. Alpha-NREM EEG sleep (i.e., intrusion of alpha waves into NREM sleep) may be absent in fibromyalgia. It may also be seen in primary sleep disorders (OSA, narcolepsy, PLMD and psychophysiologic insomnia), rheumatoid arthritis, systemic lupus erythematosus and, occasionally, in normal persons.

2. Chronic pain syndromes.
   a. Sleep-related complaints: Sleep fragmentation, EDS and fatigue.
   b. PSG features: Low sleep input pattern.

3. Juvenile rheumatoid arthritis.
   a. Seep-related complaints: EDS. Greater likelihood of OSA, RLS and PLMD.
   b. PSG features: Low sleep input pattern.

Miscellaneous disorders

1. Achondroplasia: Greater risk for OSA.
2. Down syndrome: Increased likelihood of OSA, CSA, insomnia and PLMD.
3. Prader-Willi syndrome: Increased risk of (1) OSA due to obesity, and (2) ventilatory abnormalities, including hypoventilation.
4. Sickle cell disease: Sleep disturbance during painful crises. Increased risk of OSA due to adenotonsillar hypertrophy. O_2 desaturation secondary to OSA, in turn, can result in more frequent painful crises.
5. Burns: Sleep disturbance due to pain or pruritus. EDS and nightmares are common. PSG features: Low sleep input pattern.

Neurological Disorders

In this section
Amyotrophic lateral sclerosis
Asperger disorder
Attention deficit hyperactivity disorder
Autistic disorder
Blindness
Brain injury (traumatic)
Cerebral degenerative disorders
Cerebral palsy
Dementia (Alzheimer's)
Down syndrome
Headache syndromes
Meningomyelocele
Mental retardation
Multiple sclerosis
Multiple system atrophy
Neuromuscular disorders
Parkinson disease
Progressive supranuclear palsy
Rett syndrome
Seizure disorders
Spinal cord diseases
Stroke

Amyotrophic lateral sclerosis
1. Sleep-related conditions: EDS, insomnia and SRBD (OSA and CSA). OSA is seen predominantly during REM sleep.
   a. Nocturnal O_2 desaturation may occur due to hypoventilation and diaphragmatic dysfunction.
2. Noninvasive positive pressure ventilation should be considered for patients with muscle dysfunction or SRBD.

Asperger disorder
1. Impairment in social interaction with limited patterns of activities and interests.
2. Gender: M > F.
3. Key points: Insomnia (typically with disturbed sleep in the 1st part of the night) in 90% of patients.

Attention deficit hyperactivity disorder
1. Some symptoms of inattention and hyperactivity are present prior to 7 years of age, leading to impairments at home, school or work.
2. Variable sleep-wake schedules, sleep-onset insomnia (bedtime resistance), problematic night waking, sleep fragmentation and EDS. Increased prevalence of SRBD and PLMD.
3. PSG features: Low sleep input pattern.

4. SD may exacerbate symptoms of ADHD.

Autistic disorder
1. Impaired functioning in language, social interaction, behavior or interests beginning before 3 years of age.
2. May be associated with (a) rhythmic movement disorders (e.g., head banging) continuing beyond 10 years of age, (b) insomnia, including problematic night waking, and (c) CRSD (DSPD or ISWP).

Blindness
1. Sleep-related complaints:
   a. Insomnia, problematic night waking and EDS.
   b. ↑ Prevalence of CRSD (e.g., FRD in blind persons with no light perception).
2. PSG features: ↓ TST.

Brain injury (traumatic)
1. ↑ N3 sleep (immediately after brain injury).

Cerebral degenerative disorders
1. Abnormalities in cognition, behavior and movement. Include Huntington disease, musculorum deformans, olivopontocerebellar and spinocerebellar degeneration and spastic torticollis.

2. Muscle contractions are most prominent during N1 and N2 sleep.
3. Persons with olivopontocerebellar degeneration may present with CSA, nocturnal stridor, OSA or RBD.
4. PSG features: Low sleep input pattern.

Cerebral palsy
1. ↑ Risk of OSA.

Dementia (Alzheimer's)
1. Characterized by significant, and often progressive, neurocognitive impairment.
2. Sleep-related complaints:
   a. Insomnia. EDS.
   b. OSA (↑ risk in the presence of the apolipoprotein ε4 (APOE4) allele).
   c. Reversal of day-night circadian rhythmicity.
   d. Nocturnal confusion and wandering ("sun downing").
3. PSG features:
   a. Low sleep input pattern.
   b. ↓ Sleep spindles and K-complexes.
   c. ↓ N3.
   d. ↑ REM SL and ↓ R (especially in advanced disease).
4. Note: Increased risk for RBD in persons who have dementia with Lewy bodies.

Down syndrome
1. ↑ Risk of OSA.

Headache syndromes
1. Certain headaches occur during both sleep and waking (e.g., migraine, cluster headache, and chronic paroxysmal hemicrania), and others occur only during sleep, such as hypnic headaches.
2. PSG features: Low sleep input pattern.
3. *Migraine headaches.*
   a. Episodic headaches, often unilateral, associated with nausea, vomiting, photophobia or phonophobia.
   b. An aura consisting of scintillating scotomas and homonymous visual field defects precedes a "classic migraine", but is absent in "common migraine".
4. *Cluster headaches.*
   a. Excruciating, unilateral (periorbital or temporal) headaches that occur in "clusters". During cluster periods, 1-3 headache attacks can occur daily, often at the same hour each day. Each individual attack lasts for about a few hours.
   b. Headaches may be accompanied by lacrimation, conjunctival injection, rhinorrhea or nasal stuffiness, miosis, ptosis and increased ipsilateral forehead sweating.
   c. Gender: M > F.
   d. May be triggered by OSA.
5. *Chronic paroxysmal hemicranias.*
   a. Severe unilateral headaches (e.g., temporal, orbital or supraorbital) that are responsive to therapy with indomethacin.
6. *Hypnic headache.*
   a. Generalized or unilateral headaches that occur during sleep and may be accompanied by nausea.
   b. Responds to therapy with lithium.
7. Unbelievable but true!:
   a. Migraines, cluster headaches and chronic paroxysmal hemicrania commonly have their onset during sleep.
   b. Migraine headaches can occur during N3 or REM sleep.
   c. Cluster headaches tend to occur during sleep (especially during REM sleep).
   d. Chronic paroxysmal hemicrania is most commonly associated with REM sleep.
   e. Hypnic headaches occur only during sleep (most commonly during REM sleep and, less commonly during N3 sleep).
   f. Persons with OSA may present with transient early morning headaches that occur upon awakening.

Meningomyelocele
1. ↑ Risk of UA obstruction and OSA.
2. Central apneas and hypoventilation can develop in cases associated with type II Arnold-Chiari malformation.

Mental retardation
1. Sub-average intellectual functioning.
2. Sleep-related complaints: Insomnia, sleep fragmentation, PLMS, and rhythmic movement disorder.

Multiple sclerosis
1. Sleep-related complaints: Insomnia, RBD, RLS and secondary narcolepsy.

Multiple system atrophy
1. Sleep-related conditions: RBD and SRBD.
2. Sudden death during sleep may occur due to vocal cord abductor paralysis. This

syndrome presents with nocturnal stridor, and is associated with a worse outcome. Laryngoscopy during sleep aids in diagnosis. Management, in many cases, consists of tracheotomy.

3. *Shy-Drager syndrome:* Sleep-related complaints: SRBD (OSA, CSA, CSR, apneustic breathing and inspiratory gasping), nocturnal hypoxemia, insomnia and RBD.

Neuromuscular disorders
1. Sleep-related complaints:
   a. Sleep disturbance, insomnia and EDS.
   b. ↑ Risk of OSA.
   c. ↑ Risk of nocturnal hypoventilation (O_2 desaturation is most pronounced during REM sleep). Nocturnal hypoventilation can precede abnormalities occurring during waking by months to years. The risk of sleep-related O_2 desaturation is greater if (a) maximal inspiratory pressure < 60 cm H2O, and (b) FVC < 50% of predicted.
   d. Nocturnal dyspnea.
2. PSG features: Low sleep input pattern.

Duchenne muscular dystrophy.
1. Sleep-related complaints: OSA and CSA.
2. PSG features: ↑ WASO and ↓ R.

Myasthenia gravis.
1. Sleep-related complaints: OSA and CSA. Nocturnal O_2 desaturation (predominantly during REM sleep) can develop.

Myotonic dystrophy.
1. Sleep-related conditions: EDS (most common complaint, and related to the degree of muscular impairment), sleep disruption, OSA, CSA, hypnagogic hallucinations, and hypoventilation (especially during REM sleep).

Poliomyelitis and post polio syndrome.
1. Poliomyelitis: Lower motor neuron disease that can involve the respiratory motor nuclei and give rise to dysfunction of respiratory muscles, including the diaphragm.
2. Post polio syndrome: New progressive weakness affecting respiratory, bulbar or extremity muscles that develops following poliomyelitis.
3. Sleep-related complaints: EDS, SRBD and nocturnal hypoventilation.
4. PSG features: Low sleep input pattern.

Parkinson disease
1. Characterized by the clinical triad of muscle rigidity, hypokinesia and resting tremors.
2. Sleep-related complaints:
   a. Insomnia (sleep-maintenance): Major complaint.
   b. Sleep fragmentation and EDS. Sleep attacks in 5% of affected persons.
   c. Parasomnias: RBD (15-30%), nightmares, hallucinations (20%), RLS (20%) and PLMD.
   d. SRBD (CSA, OSA and hypoventilation).
   e. Reversal of circadian day-night rhythms. Sun downing.
3. Causes of sleep disturbance:
   a. Nocturnal motor symptoms: Akinesia, dyskinesia, myoclonus and tremors.
   b. Rigidity and inability to turn over in bed.
   c. Nocturia.
   d. Painful leg cramps.
   e. Dementia and/or depression.
   f. Dopaminergic medications.
4. EDS and sleep attacks can develop 2nd to therapy with dopaminergic agents (e.g., pramipexole or ropinirole).
5. PSG features: Low sleep input pattern and ↓ R.

Progressive supranuclear palsy
1. Absence of vertical eye movement during REM sleep.
2. Sleep-related complaints: Insomnia.
3. PSG: ↑ Phasic twitching during REM sleep. ↓ REM sleep.

Rett syndrome
1. Multiple neurological deficits (psychomotor retardation, language impairment, gait disturbance, deceleration of head growth, and abnormal hand movements such as hand wringing) that develop following a period of apparently normal prenatal and perinatal (1st 5 months) development.
2. Gender: Has been diagnosed only in females.
3. Sleep-related complaints: Insomnia and problematic night waking (children).
4. PSG features: Low sleep input pattern.

Seizure disorders
1. Abnormal and stereotypic events due to abnormal cortical neuronal discharges.
2. Sleep can precipitate seizure activity. SD can increase interictal discharges.
3. 20-30% of persons have seizures only during sleep. 75% of persons have seizures

during both waking and sleep.
4. There are 2 peaks in the timing of nocturnal seizures, namely: (a) 2 hours after bedtime and (b) from 4-5 am.
5. Frequency of sleep-related seizures: N1 and N2 > N3 > R.
6. Sleep-related complaints of nocturnal seizures: Sleep disruption and EDS. Insomnia.
7. Clinical features suggestive of sleep-related seizures:
   a. History of daytime seizures.
   b. Abnormal stereotypical motor activity (e.g., tonic clonic or focal movements, automatisms or tongue biting).
   c. Unexplained abrupt awakenings.
   d. Urinary incontinence, especially if recent onset.
8. Precipitating factors for sleep-related seizures:
   a. Irregular sleep schedules.
   b. OSA (treatment of OSA may improve seizure control).
   c. SD.
9. Seizures that occur predominantly or exclusively during sleep:
   a. Benign epilepsy of childhood with centrotemporal spikes (BECT).
   b. Continuous spike waves during NREM sleep.
   c. Generalized tonic-clonic seizures on awakening.
   d. Juvenile myoclonic epilepsy.
   e. Autosomal dominant nocturnal frontal lobe epilepsy (ADNFLE).
   f. Tonic seizures.
10. Diagnosis requires an expanded EEG montage. Video-PSG may aid diagnosis. A normal EEG does not exclude the diagnosis of seizure disorder.
11. PSG features (during nights when seizures occur): Low sleep input pattern, ↓ N3, ↑ REM SL and ↓ R.

Benign epilepsy of childhood with centrotemporal spikes.
1. Also known as benign rolandic epilepsy. Most common form of partial seizure in children.
2. Hemifacial perioral numbness and focal clonic twitching of the face and mouth. Consciousness is preserved. Secondarily generalized tonic-clonic seizures may develop.
3. Onset during childhood. Benign clinical course with spontaneous resolution in

adulthood.
4. EEG: Centrotemporal spike and sharp waves.

Continuous spike waves during NREM sleep.
1. Formerly referred to as electrical status epilepticus of sleep. Seen in children.
2. EEG: Continuous and diffuse slow spike-wave complexes occurring throughout NREM sleep. Discharges decrease during REM sleep and disappear with awakening.
3. May present with or without any visible movements or clinical complaints.
4. Associated with neurocognitive and motor impairment.

Generalized tonic-clonic seizures on awakening.
1. Onset in the 2nd second decade of life. Favorable response to therapy.

Juvenile myoclonic epilepsy.
1. Consists of three seizure types: (a) myoclonic jerks, (b) generalized tonic-clonic seizures, and (c) absence seizures.
   a. Bilateral massive myoclonic jerks affecting the limbs that occur on awakening.
   b. Generalized tonic-clonic seizures can occur during sleep or on awakening.
2. Onset during adolescence.
3. EEG: Symmetric and synchronous 4-6 Hz polyspike and wave discharges.

Nocturnal frontal lobe epilepsy.
1. Dystonic-dyskinetic, choreoathetoid, or ballistic posturing and semi-purposeful activity occurring repeatedly during NREM sleep (nocturnal paroxysmal dystonia).
2. Sleep-related complaints:
   a. Abnormal behavior (e.g., sleep terrors or sleepwalking).
   b. Sleep fragmentation and frequent arousals.
   c. Vocalization and automatisms.
   d. EDS.
3. Onset during childhood.
4. EEG: No evident abnormal ictal or interictal discharges.
5. Therapy: Carbamazepine (for short-duration attacks).

Nocturnal temporal lobe epilepsy.
1. Motionless staring and automatisms (e.g., lip smacking) are common.
2. Associated with impaired consciousness and post-ictal confusion.

Spinal cord diseases
1. Sleep-related complaints: Insomnia and SRBD (especially in persons with quadriplegia).

Stroke
1. ↑ Risk of OSA and CSA.
2. Sleep-related complaints: Insomnia, EDS and altered dreams.

Psychiatric Disorders

In this section
General
Anxiety disorders
Eating disorders
Mood disorders
Personality disorders
Schizophrenia

General
1. Sleep disturbances are common in psychiatric and behavioral disorders. Conversely, sleep disturbance and SD can adversely influence the course of some psychiatric and behavioral disorders.
2. Common PSG features of psychiatric disorders: Low sleep input pattern and ↓ N3. ↓ REM SL can develop persons with depression, manic disorder, schizophrenia, eating disorder or borderline personality disorder. PSG abnormalities may persist even after clinical remission.
3. Medications used to treat psychiatric disorders may also cause significant sleep disturbance.

Anxiety disorders
1. Sleep-related complaints: Insomnia, frequent nighttime awakenings, recurring anxiety dreams or EDS.
2. PSG features: Low sleep input pattern, ↓ N3 and ↓ R.
3. Therapy: BZ, SSRI and TCA. Behavioral and relaxation therapy.
4. Acute stress disorder.
   a. Excessive anxiety developing within 4 weeks of a traumatic experience.
   b. Features: Detachment, depersonalization, re-experiencing of the traumatic event, and avoidance of factors that might lead to recall of the event.
   c. Insomnia is common.
5. Generalized anxiety disorder.
   a. Excessive anxiety of ≥ 6 months duration.
   b. Insomnia is common. Sleep disturbance should be distinguished from that due to psychophysiologic insomnia, in which anxiety is restricted primarily to sleep disturbance rather than generalized in nature.
6. Post-traumatic stress disorder.
   a. Chronic hyperarousal and anxiety associated with preoccupation and repetitive re-experiencing (e.g., flashbacks) of a severely traumatic or life-threatening event.
   b. Sleep-related complaints: Insomnia. EDS. Re-experiencing of the original traumatic event through frequent anxiety dreams, sleep terrors and nightmares. Bedtime resistance (in children).
   c. PSG features: Low sleep input pattern and ↓ R.
7. Panic disorder.
   a. Attacks of extreme anxiety or fear that begin spontaneously and without an identifiable precipitating factor.
   b. Sleep-related complaints:
      i. Recurrent episodes of nocturnal panic attacks (30%): Abrupt awakenings with immediate and sustained wakefulness and good recall of the event. Delayed return to sleep. More common during NREM than REM sleep. Can be triggered by SD.
      ii. Insomnia.
      iii. Fears of going to sleep.
   c. PSG features: May be normal. ↑ SOL and ↓ SE in some.
   d. Therapy: Behavioral therapy (e.g., relaxation) or pharmacotherapy (e.g., SSRI, TCA or BZ).

Eating disorders
1. Sleep-related complaints: Insomnia and repetitive nighttime awakenings.

Mood disorders
1. Characterized by major depressive, manic, hypomanic or mixed episodes.
2. *Major depressive episode.*
   a. Persistently depressed mood and anhedonia accompanied by significant functional impairment.

    b. Sleep-related complaints: Insomnia (most common) or EDS.
    c. PSG features: Low sleep input pattern, ↓ N3, ↓ REM SL and ↑ REM density.
3. *Manic episode.*
    a. Marked and persistent elevation of mood (irritability and euphoria).
    b. ↓ Sleep requirement.
    c. Sleep-related complaints: Insomnia.
    d. PSG features: Low sleep input pattern, ↓ N3, ↓ REM SL and ↑ REM density.
4. *Hypomanic episode.*
    a. Persistently elevated mood (less severe than manic episode).
    b. ↓ Sleep requirement.
    c. Sleep-related complaints: Insomnia.
5. *Mixed episode.*
    a. Mood that rapidly alternates between major depressive and manic episodes.
    b. ↓ Sleep requirement.
    c. Sleep-related complaints: Insomnia.

Major depressive disorder
1. ≥ 1 major depressive episode without any manic, hypomanic or mixed episodes.
2. Sleep-related complaints: Insomnia or EDS.
3. PSG features:
    a. Low sleep input pattern.
    b. ↓ N3 (particularly during the 1st NREM period).
    c. REM sleep abnormalities: ↓ REM SL and ↑ REM density.
    d. ↓ N3 and ↓ REM SL may persist during clinical remission.
4. Therapy: Antidepressant agents and psychotherapy.

Bipolar disorder
1. Can either be *bipolar 1* (≥ 1 manic, hypomanic or mixed episode +/- major depressive episode) or *bipolar 2* (≥ 1 major depressive episode plus ≥ 1 hypomanic episode, without manic and mixed episodes).
    a. Depressive phase: EDS with ↑ TST and ↓ REM SL.
    b. Manic phase: Sleeplessness and ↓ TST. ↓ Sleep requirements.
    c. Other sleep-related complaints: Nightmares.
2. Therapy: Antidepressant agents and psychotherapy with or without mood-stabilizing drugs (e.g., lithium).

Seasonal affective disorder
1. Development of depressive episodes during the fall and winter. Depression is absent during spring and summer, when some persons may experience hypomanic symptoms.
    a. Fall and winter: EDS. ↑ Sleep requirements.
    b. Spring and summer: ↓ Sleep requirements (in some).
2. Therapy: Phototherapy and, occasionally, antidepressant agents.

Atypical depression
1. Characterized by lethargy, increase in appetite, weight gain and sensitivity to rejection.
2. Sleep-related complaints: EDS.
3. PSG features: ↑ TST and ↓ REM SL.

Noteworthy:
1. EDS (and ↑ TST) is associated with (1) depressive phase of a bipolar disorder, (2) seasonal affective disorder, and (3) atypical depression.
2. ↑ Risk of developing a new major depression in persons with insomnia of ≥ 1 year duration.
3. Insomnia and sleep disturbance is directly related to severity of mood disorder in most persons. Insomnia may persist following remission of depression.
4. SD can reduce depressive symptoms (especially in persons characterized as "evening" types). SD may trigger mania in persons with bipolar disorder.

Personality disorders
1. Chronic patterns of cognition, behavior and interpersonal relationships that deviate from usual societal expectations.
2. Specific types of personality disorders:
    a. *Obsessive-compulsive disorder* – Presence of persistent intrusive and irrational thoughts (obsessions) and their related behaviors (compulsions).
    b. *Borderline disorder* – Impulsivity and instability in affect and relationships.
3. PSG features of *obsessive-compulsive* and *borderline disorders:* Low sleep input pattern and ↓ REM SL.

Schizophrenia

1. Chronic psychiatric disorder characterized by hallucinations, delusions, disorganized speech, affective flattening, limited goal-directed behavior, and restricted thought and speech production.
2. Sleep-related complaints: Insomnia, EDS, frightening dreams, polyphasic sleep periods, and reversal of day-night sleep patterns.
   a. Insomnia is common during acute psychotic decompensation, when a person may remain awake for prolonged periods.
   b. EDS can develop during (a) the waning phase of schizophrenia or (b) residual schizophrenia.
3. Conversely, sleep disruption can aggravate psychosis.
4. PSG features: Low sleep input pattern, $\downarrow$ N3 and $\downarrow$ REM SL.
   a. $\downarrow$ REM rebound after SD.
   b. $\downarrow$ TST and $\downarrow$ R during the waxing phase of the disorder. Normalize during the waning, post-psychotic and remission phases of the disorder.
   c. $\uparrow$ REM SL with successful therapy of schizophrenia.
5. Therapy involves antipsychotic medications. Clozapine and olanzapine are the most sedating of the newer antipsychotic agents. Risperidone is less sedating.
6. Acute psychotic decompensation may be heralded by worsening sleep disturbance.

Parasomnias

In this section
General
Catathrenia
Confusional arousals
Exploding head syndrome
Isolated sleep paralysis
Nightmare disorder
REM sleep behavior disorder
Sleep enuresis
Sleep-related dissociative disorders
Sleep-related eating disorder
Sleep terrors
Sleepwalking

General
1. Parasomnias are physical or experiential phenomena that occur during the sleep period. They manifest as activation of skeletal muscles or autonomic nervous system during sleep.
2. Disorders of arousal consist of confusional arousals, sleep terrors and sleepwalking.
   a. Greater prevalence in children, with onset usually from 4-6 years of age. Most cases spontaneously resolve by adolescence.
   b. Occur predominantly in N3 sleep, during the 1st third of the sleep period.
   c. Risk factors: SD, OSA and PLMD.
   d. Therapy: Sleep hygiene. Scheduled awakening (patients are awakened about 15-30 minutes before the time when parasomnia typically occurs and then allowed to return to sleep).
3. Parasomnias that generally occur during REM sleep include nightmares, REM sleep behavior disorder and isolated sleep paralysis. These parasomnias tend to occur during the 2nd half of the sleep period when REM sleep becomes relatively more common.

Catathrenia
1. Intermittent expiratory groaning or moaning during sleep (predominantly REM sleep).
2. Other features include hoarseness on waking and mild daytime fatigue (occasionally).
3. No associated respiratory distress, emotional anguish, abnormal motor activity, O_2 desaturation or cardiac arrhythmias.
4. Normal neurological and UA examinations.
5. Rare condition. Gender: M > F.

6. Chronic clinical course.
7. PSG feature: Normal sleep architecture.

Confusional arousals
1. Episodes of confusion following spontaneous or forced arousals from sleep.
2. Main clinical features:
   a. Disorientation.
   b. Inappropriate behavior (occasionally violent).
   c. Amnesia (anterograde and retrograde).
   d. Inconsolability.
   e. ↓ Vigilance and cognitive response.
   f. Minimal or no signs of fear or autonomic hyperactivity.
   g. Blunted responsiveness to questioning and other external stimuli.
3. Events can be precipitated by SD (most important risk factor).
   a. Other risk factors: Alcohol use, forced awakenings, idiopathic hypersomnia, narcolepsy, OSA, PLMD, shift work, sleep terrors and sleepwalking.
4. Most episodes last 5-15 minutes.
5. Strong familial pattern. Gender: M = F. More prevalent among children and adults < 35 years of age.
   a. Prevalence in 3-13 year age group: 16%.
   b. Prevalence in > 15 year age group: 4%.
6. Consequences include sleep disruption. Severity decreases with aging.
7. Two clinical variants:
   a. Severe sleep inertia.
   b. Sleep sex.
8. PSG features during episodes: Brief delta activity, N1 sleep, microsleep periods, or diffuse and poorly reactive alpha rhythm.
9. Therapy may consist of:

a. Avoidance of SD. Trial of sleep extension.
b. Scheduled awakenings.
c. Psychotherapy (for marked psychological distress).
d. Off-label use of TCA and BZ.

Exploding head syndrome
1. Awakening with a loud sound or sensation of explosion in the head. Can give rise to insomnia.
2. May be a variant of sleep starts.
3. Onset usually in adulthood. Gender: F > M.
4. Not associated with pain or neurological complications.

Isolated sleep paralysis
1. Persistence of REM-sleep muscle atonia during wakefulness.
2. Key features:
   a. Respiration is unaffected.
   b. Preservation of consciousness.
   c. Full recall of the event.
   d. Accompanied by hallucinations in 25-75% of affected persons.
3. Onset is generally during adolescence. Gender: M = F.
4. Risk factors include SD, irregular sleep-wake schedules and supine sleep position.
5. Other disorders associated with sleep paralysis:
   a. Narcolepsy.
   b. Familial form of sleep paralysis (occurring at sleep onset).

Nightmare disorder
1. Unpleasant and frightening dreams that often abruptly awaken the sleeper.
2. Typically occur during REM sleep in the 2nd half of the nocturnal sleep period.
   a. Nightmares developing after acute stress disorder or PTSD may occur during NREM sleep, particularly in N2 sleep.
3. Main clinical features:
   a. Full alertness and good recall of preceding dream on awakening.
   b. Delayed return to sleep.
   c. Minimal autonomic changes (no significant tachycardia and tachypnea).
4. Gender: M = F (children). M < F (adolescents and adults).
5. Onset usually at 3-6 years. Peak prevalence at 6-10 years. Generally become less frequent during adulthood. Post-traumatic nightmares can start at any age and can persist throughout life.
6. Can be precipitated by other disorders (OSA, narcolepsy or psychiatric disorders), febrile illness, medications, trauma and alcohol ingestion.
   a. Medications that can cause nightmares include amphetamines, antidepressants, antihypertensives (beta blockers), barbiturates, and dopamine agonists. Withdrawal from alcohol and REM sleep suppressants can also precipitate nightmares.
7. Frequent nightmares can lead to insomnia, EDS and anxiety.
8. PSG features: $\downarrow$ REM SL, $\uparrow$ REM density and $\uparrow$ R.
9. Therapy:
   a. Reassurance. Sleep hygiene.
   b. Behavioral therapy (image rehearsal).
   c. Psychotherapy.
   d. Trial of REM sleep suppressants for severe cases. Prazosin or neuroleptic agents in PTSD-related nightmares.

REM sleep behavior disorder
1. Abnormal "dream enacting" behavior and complex motor activity during REM sleep associated with loss of REM-related muscle atonia or hypotonia.
2. Key features:
   a. Rapid awakening and full alertness.
   b. Good dream recall.
   c. ANS activation is uncommon.
   d. Episodes are more common during the 2nd half of the nocturnal sleep period.
3. Clinical subtypes:
   a. Subclinical RBD: $\uparrow$ Muscle tone during REM sleep but without clinical features of RBD.
   b. Parasomnia overlap syndrome: Co-occurrence of RBD and disorders of arousal.
   c. Status dissociatus: Abnormal dream-related behaviors and admixture of waking, NREM and REM sleep [i.e., absence of identifiable sleep stages] during PSG.
4. Predisposing factors include aging, dementia with Lewy bodies, male gender, medications (e.g., TCA, SSRI or MAOI), multiple system atrophy, PD and stroke.
5. Increased prevalence of PLMS and narcolepsy in patients with RBD.
6. Prevalence: < 1% of the general population. Gender: M > F. More common in older

adults ($\geq$ 50 years of age).

7. Chronic and progressive course. Complications include injuries to self or bed partner, and sleep fragmentation.

8. Evaluation should include comprehensive neurological testing. PSG (with additional EMG monitoring of the upper extremities [flexor digitorum] and time-synchronized video recording) is indicated for diagnosis.
   a. PSG features: Normal sleep architecture. Some may have $\uparrow$ N3 and $\uparrow$ REM density. $\uparrow$ Muscle tone or phasic EMG activity during REM sleep. No seizure activity.
   b. MSLT: Normal SOL (EDS is uncommon).

9. MRI and SPECT of the brain: Decreased blood flow in the upper portion of the frontal lobe and pons. Decreased nigrostriatal presynatic dopamine transporter binding.

10. Therapy:
    a. Low-dose clonazepam at bedtime is effective in $\approx$ 90% of patients.
    b. Melatonin may restore REM sleep-related muscle atonia.
    c. Environmental precautions are essential.

11. Amazing facts:
    a. There is typically no history of violent or aggressive behavior during the day while awake.
    b. The eyes are closed during episodes of RBD. In contrast, eyes are open during sleepwalking.
    c. Clinical RBD eventually develops in 25% of cases of subclinical RBD.
    d. Periodic reassessment is recommended for delayed emergence of PD or other neurodegenerative disorders several years or decades after the onset of RBD.
    e. Clonazepam decreases RBD-related arousals and behaviors but does not significantly alter the elevated EMG tone during REM sleep.

Sleep enuresis
1. Recurrent involuntary voiding during sleep that occurs $\geq$ twice a week after 5 years of age.
2. Classified as primary or secondary:
   a. *Primary*: Child has never been consistently dry during sleep for 6 consecutive months.
   b. *Secondary*: Child or adult who had previously been dry for 6 consecutive months and then begins bedwetting $\geq$ twice a week for a period of $\geq$ 3 months.
3. Primary sleep enuresis:
   a. Prevalence decreases with aging.
      i. 4 years: 30%.
      ii. 6 years: 10%.
      iii. 10 years: 5%.
      iv. 15 years: 1%.
   b. Increased prevalence in children with ADHD or living in disorganized families.
   c. Spontaneous cure rate of primary sleep enuresis: 15% annually.
4. Secondary sleep enuresis:
   a. Risk factors include CHF, chronic constipation, dementia, depression, diabetes, OSA, seizures, stress, substance or medication use (alcohol, caffeine or diuretics) and urinary tract infection or pathology.
   b. Structural urinary tract pathology should be suspected if: (1) presence of daytime enuresis, (2) abnormalities in the initiation of urination, and (3) abnormal urinary flow.
5. Gender: M > F (primary childhood sleep enuresis). F > M (older adults).
6. Pathophysiology:
   a. Genetic predisposition.
   b. $\downarrow$ Arousability.
   c. $\downarrow$ Nocturnal antidiuretic hormone and vasopressin secretion.
   d. $\downarrow$ Urinary bladder capacity.
   e. Note: A child develops the ability to delay voiding in the presence of a full bladder by 18-36 months of age.
7. Evaluation commonly consists of a urinalysis and urine culture. Urologic evaluation is indicated for suspected structural urinary tract disorders.
8. PSG features: Occurs most commonly during NREM sleep in the 1st third of the night.
9. Treatment of enuresis includes bell and pad therapy (70% effective), bladder training or pharmacotherapy (desmopressin or imipramine). Drug therapy may be helpful for acute control, such as during sleepovers.

Sleep-related dissociative disorders
1. Nocturnal fugue state that develops within several minutes after an awakening.
2. Key features:
   a. Defensive, self-mutilating, sexualized or violent behavior.

b. Vocalization or ambulation.
c. Amnesia.
3. Associated features (in some):
   a. Daytime dissociative disorders.
   b. History of physical or sexual abuse.
   c. Psychiatric disorders (PTSD or anxiety disorder).
4. Gender: F > M. Onset during childhood to middle adulthood. Chronic course.

Sleep-related eating disorder
1. Repetitive bouts of eating or drinking during arousals from sleep. Arousals appear to be triggered by learned behavior rather than by real hunger or thirst.
2. Key features:
   a. Lack of, or partial, awareness of the abnormal behavior.
   b. Total or partial amnesia.
   c. Consumption of high-caloric foods or inappropriate substances.
3. Gender: F > M. Onset often during early adulthood.
4. Course is chronic and episodes often occur nightly and at any time during the sleep period.
5. Risk factors include poor sleep hygiene, primary sleep disorders (narcolepsy, OSA, PLMD and sleepwalking [most important]), stress, mood disorder and medications (e.g., zolpidem).
6. Consequences include weight gain, dyspepsia, sleep fragmentation and EDS.
7. PSG features include arousals from N3 sleep and, occasionally, from REM sleep.

Sleep terrors
1. Synonym: Pavor nocturnus.
2. Abrupt awakening with profound fear and intense autonomic discharge (tachycardia, tachypnea, sweating and mydriasis). Awakening generally occurs during N3 sleep, often in the 1st third of the night.
3. Key features:
   a. Vocalization (talking or screaming).
   b. Ambulation.
   c. Confusion.
   d. Amnesia.
4. Gender: M = F (children). M > F (adults). Onset usually during prepubertal childhood. Spontaneous resolution generally by adolescence.
5. Parasomnia overlap disorder is defined by

the co-occurrence of sleep terrors (or sleepwalking) and RBD.
6. Therapy:
   a. Avoidance of SD. Trial of sleep extension.
   b. Scheduled awakenings.
   c. Low-dose BZ.
   d. L-5-hydroxytryptamine (may be tried for children).
   e. Hypnosis.

Sleepwalking
1. Key clinical features: Ambulation, confusion, amnesia for the episode, inappropriate behavior (may give rise to violent activity), diminished arousability, and open eyes (in contrast, eyes are usually closed in RBD).
2. Most frequently occurs in stage N3 sleep, during the 1st half of the night. Occasionally, can emerge from stage N2 sleep (especially with SD).
3. Prevalence ranges from 17% (children) to 4% (adults). Peak prevalence between 8-12 years of age. Gender: M = F (children); M > F (adult cases associated with violence or injury).
4. Prevalence of childhood cases is strongly linked to family history:
   a. 20% when neither parent is affected.
   b. 40% when one parent is affected.
   c. 60% when both parents are affected.
5. In children, sleepwalking, sleep talking and night terrors commonly co-exist.
6. Precipitating factors include SD (most common risk factor), febrile states (in children), acute stress, OSA, internal or external stimuli (distended bladder or noise), and medication (psychotropic agents) or alcohol use.
7. Spontaneous resolution of childhood cases usually by puberty.
8. Pathophysiology involves disordered arousals and stage N3 sleep instability. SPECT scanning during sleepwalking demonstrates activation of thalamocingulate pathways as well as deactivation of other thalamocortical arousal systems. EEG power spectral analyses may reveal increased slow wave activity, greater N3 fragmentation and increased delta power prior to arousals.
9. Treatment consists of anticipatory scheduled awakenings or medications, such as BZ or TCAs (when cases are frequent or associated with injuries). Hypnosis.

Restless Legs and Periodic Limbs

In this section
General
Demographics
Clinical course
Classification
Risk factors
Consequences
Evaluation
PSG features of RLS
Suggested immobilization test
Differential diagnosis
Pathophysiology
Therapy
Periodic limb movements during sleep
Periodic limb movement disorder

General
1. Restless legs syndrome is a neurological disorder characterized by an urge to move, or unpleasant sensations, involving the legs (and less commonly the arms) that:
   a. Begin or worsen during periods of rest or inactivity.
   b. Are relieved transiently by movement.
   c. Are worse, or occur only, at night.
2. Among children (2-12 years of age), diagnosis requires either:
   a. Presence of all 4 adult criteria *and* description of leg discomfort in the child's own words.
   b. Presence of all 4 adult criteria *and* ≥ 2 of the following:
      i. Sleep disturbance.
      ii. RLS in parent or sibling.
      iii. PLMI of ≥ 5 per hour.
3. Useful mnemonic: *IDLE*
   Inactivity
   Discomfort
   Legs
   Evening

Demographics
1. Prevalence of 3-15% in the general population. Increased likelihood with anemia, uremia, pregnancy and aging. Prevalence is higher among Caucasians compared to Asians.
2. Gender: F > M.

Clinical course
1. Onset can occur at any age. Most common in middle-aged and older adults.
2. Chronic course.
3. 70-90% of persons have PLMS. One-third of persons with PLMS have RLS.

Classification
1. Primary (idiopathic) cases may be related to abnormalities in dopaminergic systems. Two subtypes, namely *early onset* (symptoms start before 35-45 years of age, more gradual progression of symptoms and more frequent family history of RLS) and *late onset*.
2. Secondary.

Risk factors
1. Iron deficiency anemia.
2. Uremia.
3. Pregnancy. Increased severity during 3rd trimester. Symptoms diminish or disappear following delivery.
4. Peripheral neuropathy.
5. Attention deficit hyperactivity disorder.
6. Parkinson disease.
7. Diabetes mellitus.
8. Rheumatoid arthritis.
9. Alcohol or caffeine ingestion.
10. Smoking.
11. Gastric surgery.
12. Medication use (SSRI, TCA, MAOI, lithium, antihistamines, neuroleptics and dopamine antagonists):
    a. Note: Bupropion does not cause or aggravate RLS or PLMS.

Consequences
1. Sleep-onset and sleep-maintenance insomnia. Bedtime resistance and problematic night waking in children.
2. EDS due to sleep fragmentation.

Evaluation
1. Clinical history.
2. Normal neurological examination in primary RLS.
3. Laboratory evaluation including CBC, serum iron, ferritin, folate, electrolytes, thyroid function tests, fasting glucose and renal panel.
4. PSG is not routinely indicated.
5. Suggested immobilization test.

PSG features of RLS
1. Low sleep input pattern.
2. PLMW > 15 per hour may be present prior to sleep onset.
3. PLMS may be present.

Suggested immobilization test
1. PSG is performed for 1 hour prior to habitual evening bedtime with the patient awake, sitted upright in bed and with legs outstretched. PLMW > 40 per hour supports the diagnosis of RLS.

Differential diagnosis
1. Akathisia related to the use of neuroleptic agents or dopamine receptor antagonists.
2. Peripheral neuropathy.

Pathophysiology
1. Dysregulation of dopaminergic system:
   a. ↓ Dopamine receptor binding.
   b. Presynaptic dopaminergic hypofunction.
   c. ↓ Tyrosine hydroxylase in substantia nigra.
2. Abnormal iron metabolism:
   a. ↓ Brain iron in putamen, red nucleus and substantia nigra.
   b. ↓ CSF ferritin. ↑ CSF transferritin.
   c. ↓ Serum ferritin.
   d. Impaired iron uptake and transport across blood-brain barrier.
   e. Note: Ferritin is necessary as a cofactor for tyrosine hydroxylation, a rate-limiting step in dopamine synthesis.

Therapy
1. Treatment of underlying causes or precipitating factors.

2. Iron supplementation if serum ferritin < 50 µg/L.
3. Dopaminergic agents (e.g., levodopa, pergolide, pramipexole, ropinirole and rotigotine).
   a. ↓ RLS symptoms, ↓ frequency of PLMS, and improve sleep quality.
   b. Adverse effects:
      i. Augmentation: Earlier onset or increased severity of symptoms, or involvement of other body parts such as the arms (more likely with levodopa).
      ii. Rebound: Recurrence of symptoms later in the night or early morning (more likely with levodopa).
      iii. Pramipexole and ropinirole: Nausea, sleepiness, orthostasis and development of compulsive disorder.
         1. Ropinirole: Hepatically metabolized.
         2. Pramipexole: Renally cleared.
      iv. Pergolide use has been associated with the development of pleuropulmonary and cardiac valve fibrosis.
   c. Not recommended for use in children and pregnant women.
4. Benzodiazepines (e.g., clonazepam).
   a. ↓ RLS symptoms, ↓ PLMS-related arousals and improve sleep quality.
   b. Does not reduce frequency of PLMS.
5. Opioid agents (e.g., oxycodone and propoxyphene).
   a. ↓ RLS symptoms and ↓ PLMS.
   b. May be considered for severe symptoms refractory to other therapy.
6. Other medications:
   a. Anticonvulsant agents (e.g., carbamazepine and neurontin): Neurontin may be considered for RLS accompanied by pain.
   b. Clonidine.

Periodic limb movements during sleep
1. Recurrent leg movements that commonly consists of partial flexion of the ankle, knee and hip with extension of the big toe. (*Imagine pulling back your foot and leg after stepping on a gas pedal with your toes.*) Involvement of the upper extremity consists of flexion at the elbow.
2. Can also occur while sitting or lying during restful wakefulness, referred to as periodic limb movements during wakefulness

(PLMW).

3. Prevalence of 5% in the general population. More common among middle-aged and older adults. Gender: M = F.
4. Share many of the risk factors of RLS. Disorders that are associated with PLMS include RLS (most important), narcolepsy, RBD, OSA and spinal cord injury.
5. PSG is required for diagnosing PLMS (using EMG of the anterior tibialis muscles). Diagnostic criteria:
   a. Duration of 0.5-5 seconds.
   b. Occur in a series of ≥ 4 consecutive contractions.
   c. Interval between movements of 5-90 seconds from the *onset* of one limb movement to the *onset* of the next.
   d. EMG amplitude of ≥ 25% than baseline levels noted during biocalibration.
   e. Contractions occurring simultaneously in both legs are counted as one movement.
   f. Leg movements occurring during arousals related to SRBD events are not counted.
6. Periodic limb movement index (PLMI) is the total number of PLMS per hour of TST.
   a. PLMI is abnormal if (1) > 5 in children and (2) > 15 in adults.
7. Note:
   a. There is significant night-to-night variability in PLMS frequency. PLMS are more frequent during the 1st part of the sleep period. Sleep quality may improve during the latter part of sleep.
   b. More common during NREM sleep, especially N2, than REM sleep.

Periodic limb movement disorder
1. PLMD is defined by symptomatic PLMS with complaints of sleep disturbance or EDS. The PLMI does not correlate well with degree of sleep disturbance or EDS.
2. Therapy of PLMD is similar to that of RLS. Specific therapy is not indicated for asymptomatic PLMS.

Circadian Rhythm Sleep Disorders

In this section
General
Advanced sleep phase disorder
Delayed sleep phase disorder
Free-running disorder
Irregular sleep-wake rhythm
Jet lag disorder
Shift work sleep disorder
Due to medical or neurological disorders
Therapy

General
1. Caused by a recurrent or persistent misalignment between the desired sleep schedule and the circadian sleep-wake rhythm.
2. Can be associated with insomnia or EDS (or both).

Advanced sleep phase disorder
1. Early bedtime (6-9 pm) and early wake time (2-5 am). Inability to delay sleep time. Sleep, itself, is normal for age.
2. Excessive sleepiness in the late afternoon or early evening. Morning awakening that is earlier than desired.
3. Onset is commonly during middle age. Prevalence of 1% in middle-aged and older adults. Gender: M = F.
4. Pathophysiology:
   a. Possible mechanisms include (a) shorter than normal endogenous circadian rhythm period; (b) inability to phase delay; and (c) altered homeostatic regulation of sleep.
5. Diagnosis requires sleep logs or actigraphy performed over several days. Phase advance in CTmin and DLMO. "Morning type" on the Horne-Ostberg test.
6. PSG: Normal if performed during the preferred advanced sleep time. ↓ SOL, ↓ TST and ↓ REM SL if performed during a conventional later sleep time.
7. Therapy: Early evening bright light therapy (before CTmin). Chronotherapy (gradually shifting the usual sleep time until the desired bedtime is achieved).
8. Key points:
   a. Depression, which may also present with early morning awakenings, should be excluded.
   b. The preadolescent child may have a mild degree of phase-advancement.

Delayed sleep phase disorder
1. Chronic inability to fall asleep until the early morning hours (1-6 am) and difficulty arising until late morning or early afternoon (10 am to 2 pm). In short, the major nocturnal sleep period occurs habitually later than the desired or socially acceptable bedtime.
   a. There is no difficulty remaining asleep following the onset of sleep.
   b. Occasionally, marked difficulty with awakening in the morning may be associated with confusion (sleep inertia).
2. The disorder is due to a phase delay of the circadian sleep-wake rhythm coupled with an inability to phase advance in order to correct the disturbance.
3. Onset is often during adolescence. Prevalence of 0.1-0.2% in the general population.
   a. More common among adolescents and young adults with a prevalence of 2-15% in this age group.
   b. Gender: M > F.
4. Chronic course. Severity may diminish with increasing age.
5. Diagnosis is made by history and sleep diaries.
   a. Actigraphy monitoring for ≥ 7 days reveals a stable delay of the habitual sleep period.
   b. "Evening type" score on the Horne-Ostberg chronotype scale.
   c. Delays in the timing of CTmin and DLMO are present.
   d. PSG is not routinely indicated for the diagnosis of DSPS.
6. PSG features: (1) ↑ SOL and ↓ TST when performed during desired conventional sleep-wake times; or (2) normal sleep architecture when performed during the habitually delayed sleep period.

7. Treatment
   a. *Bright light therapy* (timed early morning light exposure and evening avoidance of bright light). Light exposure should occur after CTmin, which is often about 1-2 hours after the habitual mid-sleep time.
   b. *Chronotherapy* (either progressive phase delay or progressive phase advancement of the major sleep episode until the desired bedtime is reached).
   c. *Melatonin* administered in the early evening (phase shifting effect is less potent than bright light therapy).
8. A good recall method:

   There once was a young prince from Istanbul
   Who couldn't get up early to go to school
   He stayed up all night
   But he stood upright when given day light
   And majestically declared, "That's cool!"

Free-running (non-entrained, non-24-hour sleep-wake) circadian disorder

1. Progressive daily delay in sleep-onset and wake times that result in *periodically recurring* problems of insomnia or EDS. The major sleep period progressively "marches" throughout the day, afternoon and evening.
2. FRD is due to an abnormal synchronization between the endogenous sleep-wake circadian rhythm and the 24-hour environmental light-dark cycle. Freed of exogenous entraining influences such as light, the sleep-wake pattern relies solely on free-running intrinsic biologic rhythms that behave with a periodicity of slightly over 24 hours.
3. Most affected persons are totally blind and lack photic entrainment.
   a. Among blind persons, 70% complain of chronically disturbed sleep, and 40% have recurring and cyclical insomnia.
   b. Sleep is normal in some blind persons due to a functional retinohypothalamic pathway (i.e., they demonstrate melatonin suppression with light exposure) or to entrainment to non-photic cues.
   c. May also affect sighted persons with dementia, mental retardation or psychiatric disorders.
   d. Rare in the general population.

4. Onset can occur at any age. Gender: M = F. No known familial patterns.
5. Chronic course.
6. Diagnosis is made by history and sleep diaries or actigraphy performed over several days.
   a. Progressive delays in CTmin and DLMO.
   b. PSG is not routinely indicated for diagnosis.
7. PSG features:
   a. Normal SE.
   b. Progressively longer SOL and shorter TST when PSG is recorded at a fixed period over several days.
   c. Normal sleep duration if patients are allowed to sleep *ad libitum*.
8. Treatment:
   a. Evening administration of melatonin.
   b. Bright light therapy for sighted persons or blind persons with light perception.
   c. Regular sleep-wake and daytime activity schedules.
9. Unforgettables:
   a. FRD should be considered in any blind person presenting with complaints of recurring episodes of insomnia and EDS.
   b. A neurological evaluation to exclude any CNS pathology is recommended for sighted persons with FRD.

Irregular sleep-wake rhythm

1. No stable circadian sleep-wake rhythm. Variable, inconsistent and multiple sleep and wake periods throughout the day and night, and from one day to another. Normal aggregate sleep time over a 24-hour period.
2. Persons present with insomnia or EDS.
3. Rare condition. Most frequently seen in association with neurological disorders (e.g., dementia or mental retardation). Gender: M = F.
4. Chronic course.
5. Evaluation: Clinical history, sleep diary and actigraphy.
6. Therapy: Sleep hygiene and evening administration of melatonin.
7. Important point:
   a. Sleep-wake variability is common among newborn infants and is not considered pathologic until after 6-9 months of age when consolidation of nighttime sleep occurs.

Jet lag

1. Transient insomnia or EDS following rapid eastward or westward air travel across multiple (≥ 2) time zones due to lack of synchrony to the new local time zone.
   a. Eastward flight: Sleep-onset insomnia and difficulty awakening the next day.
   b. Westward flight: Early evening sleepiness and early morning awakening.
2. Symptoms are worse (a) following eastward travel, (b) with greater amounts and rates of time zone transitions, and (c) with increasing age.
3. Course is self-limited. Symptoms remit spontaneously within approximately a day for every time zone change.
4. PSG features: ↓ SE and ↑ WASO.
   a. ↑ SOL with eastbound travel.
5. Therapy:
   a. Phototherapy.
      i. Evening bright light exposure for westward travel.
         1. For instance, for travel from New York to California, provide 30 minutes of evening light at destination.
      ii. Morning bright light exposure after eastward travel.
         1. For example, for travel from California to New York, provide 30 minutes of morning light at destination.
   b. Short-acting hypnotic agents or melatonin at bedtime for insomnia.
6. Rule of thumb: Another diagnosis (e.g., psychophysiologic insomnia) should be considered if sleep disturbance persists for > 2 weeks following air travel.

Summary of phototherapy for jet lag:
   Get what you do not already have.
   You do not need the evening city lights of New York (for eastward travel); instead, get day light.
   You do not need the sunny days of California (for westward travel); rather, get evening light.
Note: These recommendations may not be appropriate for more extensive time zone changes (e.g., travel from North America to Asia or Europe). For additional information regarding phototherapy for these travel destinations, please consult sleep medicine textbooks or online travel services.

Shift work sleep disorder

1. Sleep disturbance is directly related to non-standard work schedules, and is due to a disparity between the timing of work and the requirement for sleep.
2. About 20% of the workforce in industrialized countries is involved in some form of non-standard work schedule (rotating shifts or permanent nighttime work schedules)
3. About 10% of shift workers develop SWSD (sleepiness and decreased alertness during night shifts, insomnia during daytime sleep periods, and non-restorative sleep).
4. Factors that increase the risk of developing SWSD include: (a) aging, (b) female gender, (c) "morningness" circadian rhythm preference, and (d) backward (counterclockwise) shift rotation schedule.
5. Consequences of SWSD include:
   a. ↑ Work-related accidents.
   b. ↓ QOL.
6. Evaluation includes sleep diaries recorded over several days. Actigraphy may aid diagnosis. PSG is not routinely indicated.
7. PSG features: Low sleep input pattern.
8. Therapy involves measures that increase nighttime alertness (appropriately timed bright light exposure in the workplace; napping before, or during, night work; and administration of psychostimulants [e.g., caffeine, modafinil or armodafinil] during evening work hours).
   a. Enhancement of daytime sleep (use of hypnotics, including melatonin, prior to post-shift daytime sleep; and restricted daytime light exposure, such as using dark sunglasses, during the morning trip home from work).

Circadian rhythm sleep disorders due to medical or neurological disorders

1. Encephalopathy from liver cirrhosis.
2. Dementia.

Therapy of circadian rhythm sleep disorders

1. Fiat lux! (Let there be light).
   Sunlight for DSPD
   Moonlight for ASPD
   Sunlight for eastward flights
   Moonlight for westward flights

2. Light exposure *after* CTmin will phase *advance* circadian rhythms.*(Remember: AA: after = advance)*. Light exposure *before* CTmin will phase *delay* circadian rhythms.

3. For SWSD:
   a. Light exposure *before* CTmin for a day-to-evening-to-night rotating work schedule
   b. Light exposure *after* CTmin for a night-to-evening-to day work schedule

4. Light therapy should be complemented by appropriate light restriction at either the start or end of the sleep period.

5. Retinopathy is a contraindication to light therapy.

Short reminders

1. ASPD: *Morning lark.*
2. DSPD: *Night owl.*
3. Irregular sleep-wake disorder: *"Atrial fibrillation" of circadian rhythms (irregularly irregular rhythm).*
4. Free-running circadian disorder:
   *Three **blind** mice,*
   *three **blind** mice,*
   *see how they **"free run"** ....*
5. Jet lag: Worse symptoms with eastward travel and aging. *Therefore to minimize symptoms, remember the old adage, "Go west, young man."*

Other Disorders in a Nutshell

In this section
Alternating leg muscle activation
Benign sleep myoclonus of infancy
Environmental sleep disorder
Fragmentary myoclonus
Hypnagogic foot tremor
Hypnotic-dependent sleep disorder
Long sleeper
Propriospinal myoclonus at sleep onset
REM sleep-related sinus arrest
Rhythmic movement disorder
Short sleeper
Sleep hyperhidrosis
Sleep-related abnormal swallowing syndrome
Sleep-related bruxism
Sleep-related choking syndrome
Sleep-related laryngospasm
Sleep-related leg cramps
Sleep-related neurogenic tachypnea
Sleep-related painful erections
Sleep start
Sleep talking
Snoring
Stimulant-dependent sleep disorder
Subwakefulness syndrome
Sudden infant death syndrome
Sudden unexplained nocturnal death syndrome
Terrifying hypnagogic hallucinations
Toxin-induced sleep disorder

Alternating leg muscle activation
1. Brief activity of the anterior tibialis muscle of one leg that alternates with activity of the same muscle in the other leg. Can occur with or without arousals.
2. Rare. Most common among middle-aged adults. Gender: M > F. Episodes may be triggered by antidepressant medications. Benign course.
3. PSG features: Repetitive, alternating activation of the anterior tibialis EMG. Each EMG activation lasts between 0.1-0.5 seconds, ≥ 4 muscle activations occurring in sequence lasting from 1-30 seconds, and with < 2 seconds between activations.

Benign sleep myoclonus of infancy
1. Repetitive, brief and bilateral myoclonic jerks (involving large muscle groups, such as the trunk, limbs, or even the entire body) occurring only during sleep (predominantly during quiet sleep). Not accompanied by seizure activity or arousals.
2. Can be observed in neurologically normal infants during the 1st 6 months of life. Rare. Onset is generally during the first week of life. Gender: M = F.
3. Benign, self-limited course.
4. PSG features: Myoclonus occurs as 4-5 jerks per second, recurring every 3-15 minutes.
5. No specific therapy is necessary.

Environmental sleep disorder
1. Sleep complaints (insomnia, EDS or parasomnia) that are directly due to adverse environmental factors, such as excessive noise.
2. Sleep disturbance is more common among older adults, and is more apparent during the 2nd half of the sleep period.
3. PSG features:
   a. If PSG is performed in the sleep laboratory: Normal sleep architecture and sleep duration.
   b. If PSG is performed in the usual sleep

environment: Low sleep input pattern.
4. Treatment consists of removal of the offending agent/s.

Fragmentary myoclonus
1. Episodes of asynchronous and asymmetric twitch-like contractions of the muscles of the face, trunk and extremities that last from 10 minutes to over an hour.
2. May accompany OSA, CSA, hypoventilation syndromes, narcolepsy, insomnia, PLMD, RLS and Niemann-Pick (type C) disease.
3. Rare. Gender: M > F.
4. Onset is generally during adulthood. Benign course.
5. Generally asymptomatic (many cases are merely an incidental EMG finding during PSG), but can give rise to sleep disturbance and EDS.
6. PSG features:
   a. > 5 brief EMG discharges per minute.
   b. No EEG abnormalities.

Hypnagogic foot tremor
1. Rhythmic tremors of the feet or toes that occur during the wake-sleep transition or during stages N1 or N2 sleep.
2. More common among middle-aged adults. Gender: M = F.
3. May be a normal phenomenon, but can result in sleep-onset insomnia or sleep disruption if severe.
4. PSG features: Recurrent trains of 1-2 Hz leg or foot EMG potentials lasting 10-15 seconds.

Hypnotic-dependent sleep disorder
1. Sleep disturbance related to habitual use of hypnotic agents.
   a. Development of insomnia during abrupt drug withdrawal.
   b. Residual EDS following use of long-acting medications.
   c. BZ may precipitate or aggravate snoring or OSA.

Long sleeper
1. Sleep time is substantially longer than typical for the person's age group (ie, > 10 hours for a young adult). EDS develops if TST is less than the required amount of sleep.
2. Onset during childhood. Chronic course.
3. Diagnosis is aided by sleep logs or actigraphy.
4. PSG features: Normal SE and ↑ TST.

5. MSLT is normal following usual amount of nighttime sleep prior to testing.

Propriospinal myoclonus at sleep onset
1. Spontaneous muscle jerks that occur during the transition from wake to sleep and that disappear at sleep onset. Myoclonus starts in the abdominal and truncal muscles and spread slowly rostrally and caudally.
2. Rare disorder. Gender: M > F.
3. No known etiology.
4. Onset during adulthood. Chronic course.

REM sleep-related sinus arrest
1. Recurrent episodes of sinus arrest, with periods of asystole lasting up to 9 seconds in duration occurring during REM sleep.
2. Most patients are asymptomatic (palpitations or vague chest pain may occasionally be present) and do not have any cardiac pathology. Daytime ECG and coronary angiography is generally normal.
3. Episodes are not associated with arousals or SRBD.
4. Rare condition.
5. Therapy is not generally indicated.

Rhythmic movement disorder
1. Repetitive, stereotypic and rhythmic movements occurring during sleep onset and light sleep. If frequent, can give rise to sleep-onset insomnia.
2. Includes head banging, head rolling, body rolling and body rocking.
3. Body rocking is more frequent in young children (≈ 1 year of age), whereas head banging and head rolling are more common among older children.
4. Prevalence of 60% (9 months of age), < 50% (18 months of age), and 10% (4 years of age). Adult cases may be associated with autism, mental retardation or significant psychopathology. Gender: M > F.
5. Risk factors include stress and lack of environmental stimulation (e.g., child abuse or neglect).
6. Spontaneous resolution with aging. Behavioral therapy and BZ may be considered for refractory cases.
7. PSG features: 0.5-2 movements per second lasting < 15 minutes. Frequency of movements: N1 > N2/N3 > R.

Short sleeper
1. Habitual sleep duration of ≤ 5 hours daily despite voluntary attempts to lengthen sleep duration. Normal sleep onset, quality, continuity and consolidation. No impairment in daytime functioning.
2. Onset often during early adolescence or young adulthood. Gender: F > M.
3. Chronic lifelong course.
4. PSG features: ↓ SOL and ↓ TST.
5. Normal MSLT.
6. No specific therapy is necessary.

Sleep hyperhidrosis
1. Profuse sweating that occurs during sleep.
2. May be related to OSA, febrile illness or pregnancy.
3. Can lead to frequent awakenings and sleep fragmentation.

Sleep-related abnormal swallowing syndrome
1. Pooling of saliva in the oral cavity during sleep due to abnormal swallowing mechanisms.
2. Arousals from sleep due to coughing and choking.
3. A "gurgling" sound can be heard preceding each coughing spell.
4. Rare condition. Clinical course is unknown.

Sleep-related bruxism
1. Repetitive grinding or clenching of the teeth during sleep.
2. Risk factors include stress, anxiety, use of psychoactive medications (SSRI, antipsychotics and amphetamine), recreational drugs, alcohol or caffeine, smoking, cerebral palsy, mental retardation and, possibly, dental disease (e.g., malocclusion or mandibular malformation). Certain primary sleep disorders, such as OSA, RLS and RBD, are also associated with an increased likelihood of sleep bruxism.
3. Prevalence is highest during childhood and decreases with aging:
   a. Children: 16%.
   b. Adolescents and young adults: 12%.
   c. Middle-aged adults: 8%.
   d. Older adults: 4%.
4. Gender: M = F. Onset commonly during the 1st and 2nd decades of life. Strong familial tendency with 20-50% of persons having a family member with a history of bruxism.
5. Pathophysiology appears to involve a microarousal event associated with an exaggerated form of oromotor masticatory muscle activity.
6. Consequences include abnormal dental wear and damage, periodontal tissue injury, facial or jaw pain (including TMJ syndrome), headaches and unpleasant noises that might disrupt the bed partner's sleep.
7. Diagnosis requires a *current* history of witnessed teeth grinding or jaw clenching during sleep *and* evidence of tooth wear.
8. PSG features:
   a. Overall sleep architecture is normal.
   b. Episodic increases in EMG tone of the chin and masseter muscles (occurring every second and lasting for ≥ 0.5-15 seconds).
      i. ≥ 4 episodes per hour of sleep, *or*
      ii. ≥ 25 individual muscle bursts per hour of sleep, *and*
      iii. ≥ 2 audible bruxism episodes per night.
   c. May appear as artifacts on the EEG or EOG channels that are referenced to the masseter or auricular electrodes.
   d. Episodes are more common during N1 and N2 sleep compared to REM sleep. Large night-to-night variability in severity.
   e. Episodes may be associated with arousals.
   f. No abnormal EEG activity, such as seizures.
9. Therapy includes intra-oral splint devices, short-term pharmacotherapy (e.g., BZ, muscle relaxants or local administration of botulinum toxin in the masseter muscles) and behavioral therapy, such as muscle relaxation exercises.
   a. When episodes are related to OSA, successful treatment of the latter may eliminate sleep bruxism.

Sleep-related choking syndrome
1. Abrupt awakenings with a choking sensation or inability to breathe accompanied by fear and anxiety.
2. No stridor.
3. Can give rise to insomnia or sleep fragmentation.
4. Rare disorder. It is most often seen during early to middle adulthood. Gender: F > M.

Sleep-related laryngospasm
1. Acute breathlessness due to total or near-total cessation of airflow while asleep that

is followed by a sudden awakening accompanied by inspiratory stridor. Associated features include temporary hoarseness and cyanosis. Episodes last from several seconds to several minutes.
2. May be due to vocal cord spasm or tracheal swelling.
3. Probably rare. Most prevalent among middle-aged adults. Gender: M > F.

Sleep-related neurogenic tachypnea
1. Sustained tachypnea that develops during sleep.
2. May lead to sleep fragmentation and EDS.
3. Rare condition.

Sleep-related painful erections
1. Painful penile erections occurring during REM sleep.
2. No apparent penile disorder. No pain during sexual erections while awake.
3. Associated sleep complaints: Sleep-maintenance insomnia.

Sleep-related leg cramps
1. Sleep disturbance due to painful spasms or tightening of the muscles of the calf or foot. Frequent leg cramps can result in insomnia or EDS.
2. Leg cramps are relieved by forcible dorsiflexion of the foot or by local massage.
3. Risk factors include aging, dehydration and electrolyte imbalance, endocrine disorders, exercise (vigorous), oral contraceptive use, PD and pregnancy.
4. Diagnosis is based on clinical history.
5. PSG, if performed, shows an awakening that coincides with non-periodic bursts of high frequency EMG activity in the gastrocnemius muscle.

Sleep start
1. Synonym: Hypnic jerk.
2. Sudden muscle contraction of part or all of the body that occurs at sleep onset. Can involve (a) a single, brief body jerk accompanied by a sensation of "falling"; (b) flashes of light or vivid imagery; (c) loud sound; or (d) somesthetic (floating) sensation.
3. Occurs in 60-70% of the general population. Affects all age groups. Gender: M = F.
4. Precipitating factors include SD, stress, excessive caffeine ingestion, stimulant use, or intense physical activity close to bedtime.
5. PSG features: Arousal or awakening from drowsiness or N1 sleep accompanied by brief EMG potentials.
6. Course is generally benign and commonly requires no therapy.

Sleep talking
1. Synonym: Somniloquy.
2. Vocalization during sleep. Occurs in all sleep stages.
3. Gender: M = F (children), M > F (adults).
4. Precipitating factors include SD, OSA, RBD, sleep terrors, confusional arousals, sleepwalking, SRED, stress, and febrile illness.
5. No apparent clinical or psychological consequences.

Snoring
1. Production of sound during sleep due to vibration of the UA structures.
2. Prevalence: 10-12% (children), 20-40% (middle-aged adults) and 40-60% (older adults). Gender: M > F (prevalence may increase during pregnancy). OSA is present in about 25-95% of snorers.
3. Risk factors consist of obesity, positive family history, SD, supine sleep position, nasal obstruction, and medication (muscle relaxants, opioids or BZ), tobacco, alcohol and substance use.
4. PSG is not routinely indicated for diagnosis (however, may be considered when UA surgery is being considered).
5. PSG features: Snoring is often loudest during stage N3 sleep and diminishes during REM sleep. Not associated with arousals, O_2 desaturation, apneas-hypopneas, hypoventilation, or significant cardiac arrhythmias.
6. Treatment includes avoidance of precipitating factors.
    a. Non-supine sleep posture if snoring occurs exclusively or predominantly during a supine sleep position.
    b. Use of earplugs for the bed partner.
    c. Nasal or UA surgery.
    d. Oral devices.

Stimulant-dependent sleep disorder
1. Insomnia or EDS related to the use or discontinuation, respectively, of stimulant medications.

Subwakefulness syndrome
1. Subjective sensation of constant EDS without objective evidence of sleepiness. No history of frequent napping.
2. Normal PSG and MSLT findings.
3. Rare condition. Course is chronic.

Sudden infant death syndrome
1. Abrupt, unexpected death in an apparently healthy infant. Cause of death remains undetermined even after comprehensive history, postmortem examination and death scene investigation.
2. Occurs predominantly prior to 6 months of age.
3. Prevalence of 0.06% in infants between 1 month and 1 year of age. Gender: M > F.
4. Risk factors include (a) prematurity, (b) prone sleeping position, (c) pre- and postnatal exposure to tobacco smoke, (d) maternal substance abuse, (e) multiple births, (f) teenage pregnancy, (g) siblings with SIDS, (h) lower socioeconomic status, and (i) occurrence of apnea of infancy.
5. Prevention consists of having infants sleep on their back.

Sudden unexplained nocturnal death syndrome
1. Sudden death occurring during sleep without any apparent cause.
2. Mostly affects healthy adult Southeast Asian males between the ages of 25-44 years.
3. Victims have been described to display moaning, screaming, violent motor activity, or labored breathing for a few minutes prior to death.
4. Unknown pathogenetic mechanisms. Mutation in the SCN5A gene is present in some families with SUNDS.

Terrifying hypnagogic hallucinations
1. Nightmares occurring at sleep onset.
2. Sudden awakening is accompanied by intense fear, full alertness and vivid dream recall.
3. Rare condition. Benign course.

Toxin-induced sleep disorder
1. Insomnia or EDS due to CNS excitation or depression, respectively, from chronic exposure to toxins (heavy metals or chemicals).

Medicolegal Topics

In this section
Obstructive sleep apnea
Sleep-related violence

Obstructive sleep apnea

1. ↑ Risk of car accidents (particularly severe crashes) in sleepy persons with OSA. Risk is increased further with concurrent alcohol ingestion. Effective therapy of OSA decreases this risk.
2. Many persons with OSA misperceive the severity of their sleepiness (i.e., poor correlation between subjective measures and objective tests of sleepiness).
3. A history of near-miss accidents predicts future risk of car accidents.
4. Subjective or objective tests of sleepiness (e.g., MSLT or MST), AHI, degree of O_2 desaturation, and performance on driving simulation tests do not consistently and reliably predict the risk of car accidents.
5. Results of driving simulation testing include:
   a. ↑ Frequency of crashes.
   b. ↑ Tracking errors.
   c. ↑ Frequency of lapses in attention.
6. Recommendations:
   a. Regularly ask about history of drowsy driving and sleepiness-related accidents or near-miss accidents.
   b. Counsel regarding sleep hygiene, including obtaining an adequate amount of sleep. Consider a trial of sleep extension.
   c. Instruct to avoid driving whenever drowsy.
   d. Avoidance of alcohol and hypnotic agents if driving is anticipated.
   e. Assess adherence to PAP therapy.
   f. Consider MSLT and/or MWT when in doubt about degree of sleepiness.
   g. Consider a trial of modafinil for objectively-determined residual sleepiness despite PAP therapy.
   h. Schedule periodic follow-up.
   i. Consider reporting the patient with EDS due to OSA to appropriate authorities, especially if:
      i. History of severe car accidents related to unexplained or untreated EDS.
      ii. Prompt therapy for OSA cannot be provided.
      iii. Patient refuses, or is consistently non-adherent with, therapy for OSA.
      iv. Patient fails to restrict driving until OSA has been adequately controlled.
      v. Such situations are considered reportable based on local laws.

Sleep-related violence

1. There are 3 subgroups of nocturnal violent activity, namely (a) self-inflicted injuries; (b) injury to others; and (c) both.
2. Sleep disorders associated with sleep-related violence include:
   a. Confusional arousals.
   b. Medication and substance use.
   c. REM sleep behavior disorder.
   d. Sleep terrors.
   e. Sleep-related seizures.
   f. Sleepwalking.
   g. Sun downing.
3. Overall prevalence of sleep-related violence is unknown.
4. Predisposing factors for sleep-related violence include:
   a. Disturbances in wake/sleep schedules.
   b. Dysfunctional families.
   c. Male gender.
   d. History of physical or sexual abuse.
   e. Stress.
   f. Substance abuse: Drugs and alcohol.
5. Differential diagnosis:
   a. Dissociative and fugue states.
   b. Drug-related states.
   c. Intentional homicide.
   d. Malingering.
   e. Munchausen by proxy.
   f. Trance states.
   g. Volitional waking behavior.
6. Evaluation:
   a. Extensive neurological, psychiatric or neuropsychological assessment. Most persons have no underlying psychopathology.
   b. Polysomnography. In suspected seizures, may need full scalp EEG.
   c. Wake and sleep EEGs. Non-attended ambulatory EEG in home environment.
   d. Video-telemetry or simple family home video recordings.

7. Therapy:
   a. Avoidance of known facilitating and triggering factors.
   b. Proper sleep/wake hygiene.
   c. Avoidance of SD.
   d. Measures to avoid injury. *"Protect yourself and others from you."*

Main Differences in Sleep Disorders

In this section
Nightmares vs. sleep terrors vs. PTSD vs. RBD
Obstructive apneas vs. central apneas
Central sleep apnea vs. Cheyne Stokes respiration
Adult OSA vs. pediatric OSA
Narcolepsy vs. idiopathic hypersomnia

Nightmares vs. sleep terrors vs. PTSD vs. RBD

1. *Nightmares.*
   a. Time of night: Latter half of the night.
   b. Sleep stage: REM sleep.
   c. Level of consciousness: Awake and alert.
   d. Memory of episode: Full recall.
   e. Subsequent return to sleep: Delayed.
2. *Sleep terrors.*
   a. Time of night: First half of the night.
   b. Sleep stage: N3 sleep.
   c. Level of consciousness: Confused and disoriented.
   d. Memory of episode: Partial or complete amnesia.
   e. Subsequent return to sleep: Rapid.
3. *Post-traumatic stress disorder.*
   a. Time of night: Repetitive.
   b. Sleep stage: Both NREM and REM sleep.
   c. Level of consciousness: Awake.
   d. Memory of episode: Good recall.
   e. Subsequent return to sleep: Variable.
   f. Note: Associated with dreams of the traumatic event.
4. *REM sleep behavior disorder.*
   a. Time of night: Latter half of the night.
   b. Sleep stage: REM sleep.
   c. Level of consciousness: Asleep.
   d. Memory of episode: Variable.
   e. Note: Seemingly purposeful and frequently violent behavior.

Obstructive apneas vs. central apneas

1. *Obstructive apneas.*
   a. Oxygen desaturation: More severe.
   b. Hemodynamic changes: Greater.
   c. Respiratory effort: Present.
2. *Central apneas.*
   a. Oxygen desaturation: Less severe.
   b. Hemodynamic changes: Less.
   c. Respiratory effort: Absent.

Central sleep apnea vs. Cheyne Stokes respiration

1. *Central sleep apnea.*
   a. Nadir of O_2 desaturation: Following termination of apnea.
   b. Timing of arousals: Termination of apnea.
   c. Cycle time: Shorter (< 45 seconds).
   d. Period of hyperpnea: Shorter.
2. *Cheyne Stokes respiration.*
   a. Nadir of O_2 desaturation: More delayed.
   b. Timing of arousals: Peak of hyperpnea.
   c. Cycle time: Longer (> 45 seconds).
   d. Period of hyperpnea: Longer.

Adult OSA vs. pediatric OSA

1. *Adult OSA.*
   a. Excessive sleepiness: More frequent.
   b. Hyperactivity and restlessness: Less common.
   c. Usual cause/s: Obesity and/or narrow oropharynx.
   d. Gender: M > F.
   e. PSG features: Significant sleep disruption.
   f. O_2 desaturation: Greater.
   g. Respiratory event-related arousals: More frequent.
   h. Primary therapy: PAP.
2. *Pediatric OSA.*
   a. Excessive sleepiness: Less frequent.
   b. Hyperactivity and restlessness: More common.
   c. Usual cause: Adenotonsillar enlargement.
   d. Gender: M = F.
   e. PSG features: Less sleep disruption.
   f. O_2 desaturation: Less.
   g. Respiratory event-related arousals: Less frequent.
   h. Primary therapy: Adenotonsillectomy.

Narcolepsy vs. idiopathic hypersomnia

1. *Narcolepsy.*
   a. Cataplexy: May be present.
   b. Sleep paralysis and sleep hallucinations: May be present.
   c. Daytime napping: Transiently refreshing.
   d. Nighttime sleep: Sleep disturbance common. ↓ SOL. ↓ REM SL.
   e. Multiple sleep latency test: ↓ SOL. SOREMPs present.
   f. HLA typing: DQB1*0602.
   g. CSF hypocretin: Low levels (narcolepsy with cataplexy). Normal levels (in some cases of narcolepsy without cataplexy).
   h. Response to stimulant therapy: More predictable improvement.

2. *Idiopathic hypersomnia.*
   a. Cataplexy: Absent.
   b. Sleep paralysis and sleep hallucinations: May be present.
   c. Daytime napping: Not refreshing.
   d. Nighttime sleep: May be normal or prolonged in duration.
   e. Multiple sleep latency test: ↓ SOL. SOREMPs may be present.
   f. HLA typing: CW2.
   g. CSF hypocretin: Normal levels.
   h. Response to stimulant therapy: Less predictable improvement.

90 Things a Somnologist Should Know

1. Indications for PSG.
2. Key clinical features of RLS in adults and children.
3. Non-pharmacologic cognitive behavioral therapies for insomnia.
4. Treatment of persistent sleepiness in OSA despite PAP therapy.
5. Complex sleep apnea.
6. Scoring rules for PLMS.
7. Distinguishing features of sleep terrors, nightmares and nocturnal panic attacks.
8. Countermeasures for sleepiness in SWSD.
9. Gender differences in the prevalence and presentation of sleep disorders.
10. Congenital central alveolar hypoventilation syndrome.
11. Nocturnal seizures.
12. Pharmacologic therapy of comorbid insomnia.
13. Afferent and efferent pathways of the circadian neurosystem.
14. PSG artifacts and their corrective measures.
15. Management of RBD and other violent sleep-related behaviors.
16. Developmental milestones in sleep physiology, architecture and behavior in children.
17. Changes in physiologic processes associated with insomnia.
18. Treatment of OSA in children and adults.
19. Treatment of the different parasomnias.
20. Ventilatory support for persons with hypoventilation syndromes.
21. Differences between CSR and CSA.
22. Light therapy for jet lag and other circadian rhythm sleep disorders.
23. Disorders that can predispose to RBD.
24. Retinal photoreceptors involved with circadian entrainment and the effects of different light wavelengths on them.
25. Mood disorders and their effects on sleep.
26. Distinguishing features of the various circadian rhythm sleep disorders.
27. Disorders of arousal.
28. Countermeasures for sleepiness.
29. Medico-legal aspects of OSA.
30. EEG, EOG and EMG electrode placements during PSG.
31. Obesity hypoventilation syndrome.
32. Clinical features of paradoxical insomnia.
33. Treatment of nightmares with image rehearsal.
34. EEG waveforms.
35. Changes in sleep architecture with alcohol use and withdrawal.
36. Actigraphy.
37. Neurotransmitters and their corresponding neural systems.
38. Distinguishing hypocapnic and hypercapnic central sleep apnea.
39. Causes (including medications) of sleep-related eating disorder.
40. Clinical course of rhythmic movement disorder.
41. Clinical course of Kleine Levin syndrome.
42. Consequences of sleep deprivation.
43. Effects of aging on sleep physiology and sleep disorders.
44. Treatment of RLS and PLMD.
45. Scoring adult, pediatric and infant sleep stages.
46. Multiple system atrophy.
47. Respiratory patterns during sleep in infants and adults.
48. Fatal familial insomnia.
49. Measuring respiration and ventilation during sleep.
50. Therapy of nocturnal enuresis.
51. Sleeping sickness.
52. How to perform MSLT and MWT.
53. ECG features of atrial fibrillation, wide complex tachycardia, and narrow complex tachycardia.
54. Exploding head syndrome.
55. Medications that may precipitate or worsen RLS or PLMD.
56. Scoring rules for adults and pediatric respiratory events.
57. Leg cramps.
58. Overlap syndrome.
59. Sleep-related disorders in Parkinson disease and dementia.
60. Nocturnal asthma.
61. Measures to improve adherence to PAP therapy.
62. Indications for oral devices for the therapy of OSA.
63. Treatment of high-altitude periodic breathing.
64. Differential diagnosis of nocturnal

oxygen desaturation.
65. Likelihood ratios, confidence intervals and number needed to treat.
66. P_{CRIT}.
67. Thermoregulation during sleep.
68. Effect of cytokines on sleep.
69. Zeitgebers.
70. Melatonin: synthesis and receptors.
71. CTmin and DLMO.
72. Evaluation of nocturnal gastroesophageal reflux.
73. Indications and limitations of APAP.
74. Management of sleep-onset central apneas.
75. Scoring arousals during NREM vs. REM sleep.
76. Extinction techniques for childhood insomnia.
77. Sleep-related headache syndromes.
78. Epworth sleepiness scale.
79. Genetics of narcolepsy.
80. Differential diagnosis of excessive sleepiness.
81. Adaptive servo ventilation.
82. Management of sleep bruxism.
83. Use of melatonin and light therapy in circadian rhythm sleep disorders.
84. Adverse effects of chronic benzodiazepine use.
85. Mammalian circadian genes.
86. American Academy of Sleep Medicine Standards of Practice guidelines.
87. Therapy of behavioral insomnias of childhood.
88. Ventilatory loop gain.
89. Managing simple snoring.
90. Causes of comorbid insomnia.

Epochs and Tracings

Stage Wake.

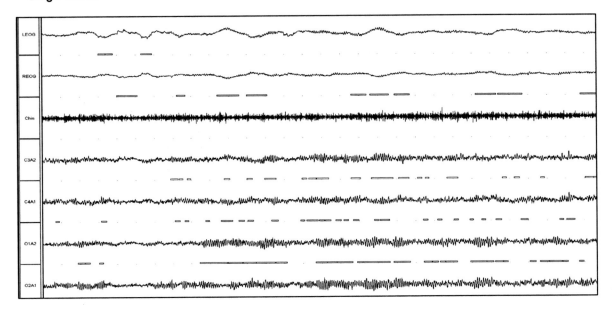

Stage N1.

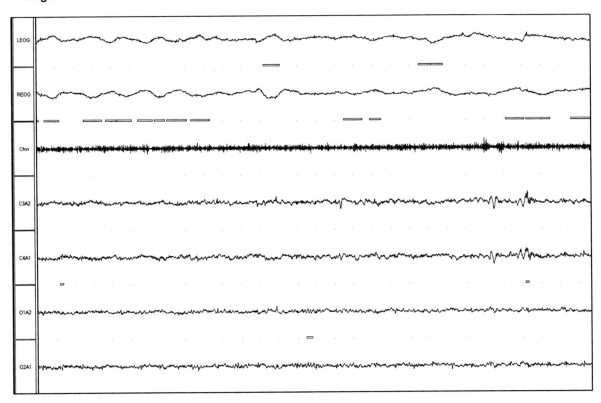

Stage N2.

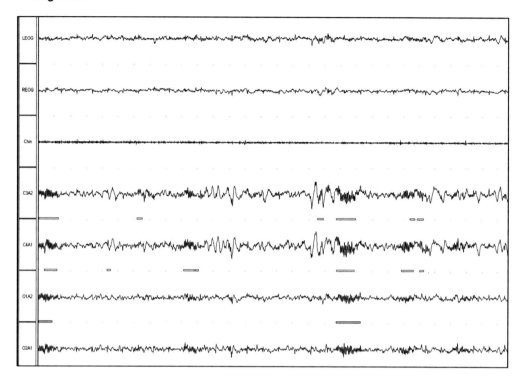

Stage N3.

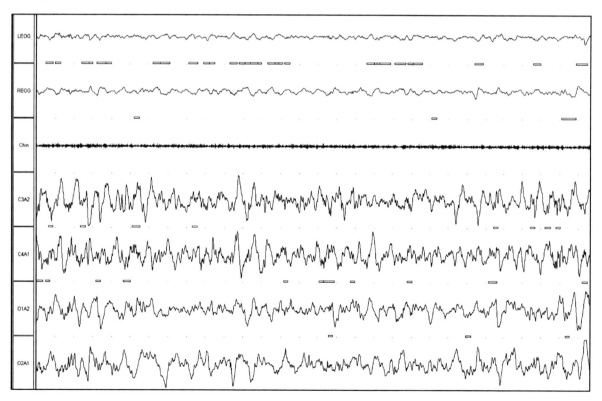

Stage REM.

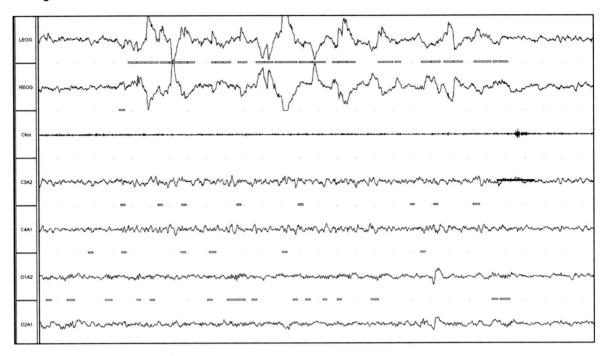

Obstructive apnea.

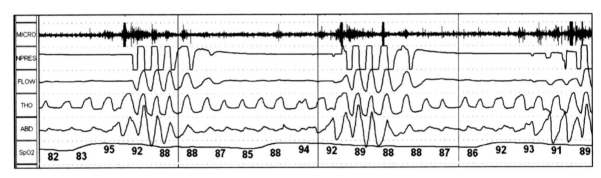

Mixed apnea.

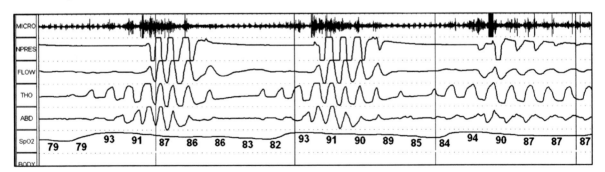

Hypopnea.

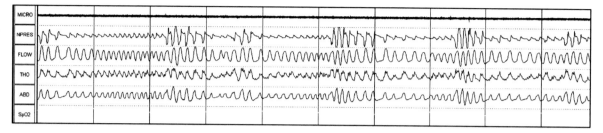

Respiratory effort-related arousal.

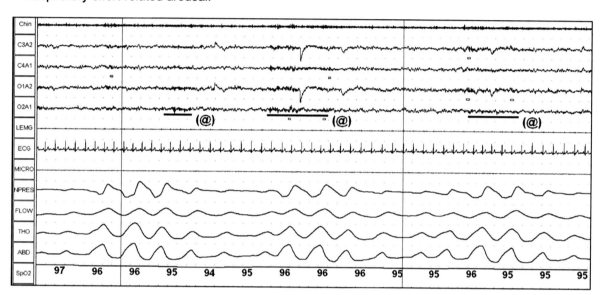

Central apnea.

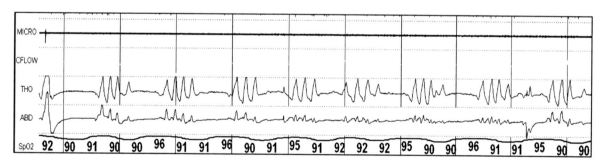

Cheyne Stokes respiration.

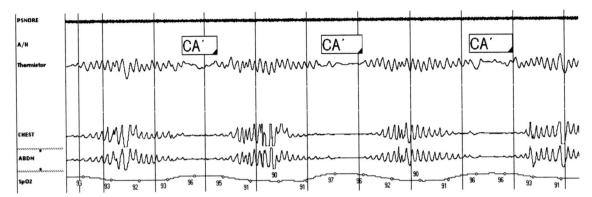

Sweat artifact.

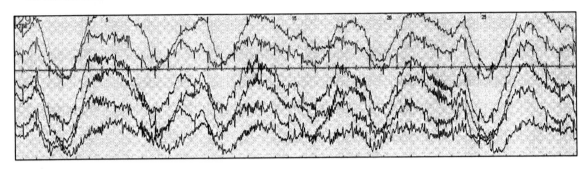

Electrode popping.

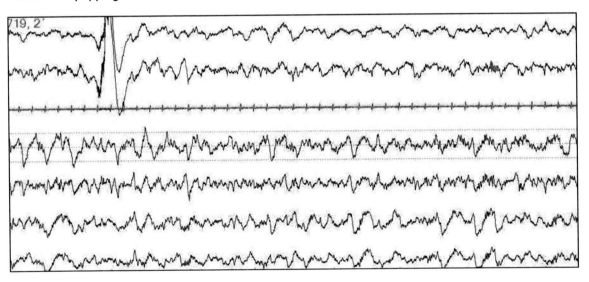

60 Hz artifact.

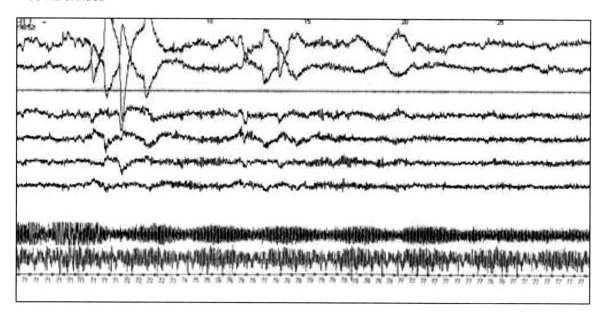

Bruxism.

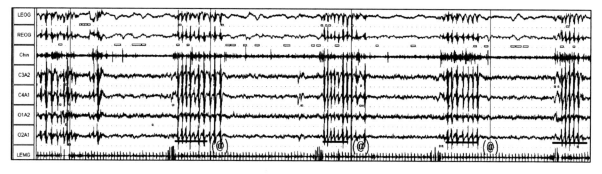

EMG artifact.

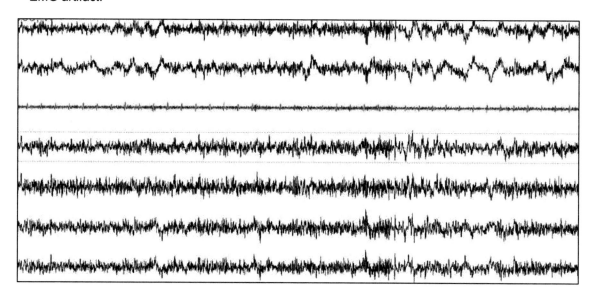

Seizure activity.

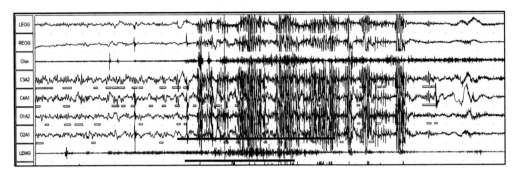

Wide-complex tachycardia.

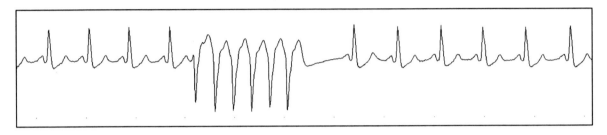

Atrial fibrillation.

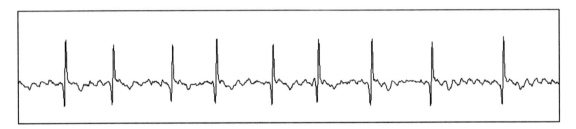

A Final Word

Test taking is a skill that can be learned. When in doubt about the correct answer, remember these useful caveats [which you can use at your own peril]:

Lee-Chiong's 8-fold path to test taking perfection

1. Nature abhors absolutism. Reject statements that contain the words "never" or "always".
2. On the other hand, certain words make any statement almost always true; these include "may", "might" and "can".
3. Exceptions are rarely the rule in nature – among several averages, choose the one closest to the mean.
4. It is often more difficult for an examiner to make up wrong statements than it is to create true ones. When a statement sounds strange [or new] to you, it's more likely to be wrong.
5. An examination tests what you ought to know [and probably have read some time ago but have since forgotten]. Trust your instincts – the first guess is almost certainly better than your second.
6. The examiner is not out to trick you. If a question appears too easy, don't become paranoid. Instead, count your blessings and move on to the next question.
7. An "all of the above" choice is more likely to be the correct answer rather than "none of the above".
8. In my *personal* test taking experience, there is a greater probability of an "a" statement being correct and either a "c" or "d" choice to be wrong. And don't ask me why this is the case. Use this advice only as a last resort.

References

1. Lee-Chiong T. Sleep Medicine: Essentials and Review. Oxford University Press, 2008.
2. Lee-Chiong TL (ed). Sleep: A Comprehensive Handbook. John Wiley & Sons, Hoboken, New Jersey, 2006.
3. Lee-Chiong TL, Sateia M, Carskadon M (eds). Sleep Medicine. Hanley & Belfus Elsevier, Philadelpha, 2002.
4. Berry RB. Sleep Medicine Pearls [2nd Edition]. Hanley & Belfus, Philadelpha. 2002.
5. Chokroverty S. Clinical Companion to Sleep Disorders Medicine Second Edition. Butterworth-Heinemann. 2000.
6. Reite M, Ruddy J, Nagel K. Concise Guide to Evaluation and Management of Sleep Disorders, Third Edition. American Psychiatric Publishing. April 2002.
7. Barkoukis TJ. Review of Sleep Medicine. Butterworth-Heinemann. 2002.
8. Lavie P, Pillar G, Malhotra A. Sleep Disorders Handbook. Taylor & Francis. 2002.
9. Perlis ML, Lichstein KL (eds). Treating Sleep Disorders: Principles and Practice of Behavioral Sleep Medicine. John Wiley & Sons, Hoboken, New Jersey, 2003.
10. Sleep Research Society. SRS Basics of Sleep Guide. Sleep Research Society. 2005.
11. Rechtschaffen A, Kales A. A Manual of Standardized Terminology, Techniques and Scoring System for Sleep Stages of Human Subjects. Brain Information Service/Brain Research Institute. University of California. 1968.
12. American Academy of Sleep Medicine. The International Classification of Sleep Disorders, Second Edition: Diagnostic and Coding Manual. American Academy of Sleep Medicine. 2005.
13. Iber C, Ancoli-Israel S, Chesson A, and Quan SF for the American Academy of Sleep Medicine. The AASM Manual for the Scoring of Sleep and Associated Event Rules: Terminology and Technical Specifications, 1st ed: Westchester, Illinois: American Academy of Sleep Medicine, 2007.

Disclosure

No one is perfect – and certainly *not* this author. Every effort has been made to verify the accuracy of the facts in this book. Any errors that were missed will be incorporated in future editions. In the meantime, kindly accept my sincere apology if any correction has been overlooked or if any concept has not been satisfactorily presented.

Airport Blues

A major part of this book was written while in transit – in an airport, plane or hotel room – on small pieces of paper that I then stuffed into my wallet. When sitting became uncomfortable, I would remove the paper pieces from my wallet and try to make sense of them. Here, then, is a chronicle of ideas that had emerged over a 10-year period of travel.

Leptin and ghrelin
Leptin = lean. Ghrelin = gain.
LL-GG (lower leptin, greater ghrelin) seen in SD.

Thermoregulation
Cool down to sleep sound. Heat up to wake up.

Insomnia
I once met a man who claimed to have never slept.
 And to prove his point,
 he shared with me a diary that he had kept.
There it was – night after night of sleepless activity it seems:
 Cooking and reading and mopping;
 he even went to the gym.
He did so much from his nightly chores, he stated
 He had nothing left to do in the day but go to bed.
He would put on his pajamas at the crack of dawn
 And close his eyes till two past noon.
The first thing he'll do the minute he got out of bed
 Is to make a list of things to do for the night ahead.

Cognitive-behavioral treatments for insomnia
Avoid alcohol – *"You might feel good, but you will feel worse."*
Cognitive therapy – *"Many of the things you think you know about your sleep are wrong."*
Paradoxical intention - *"I dare you to try to stay awake."*
Relaxation techniques - *"Relax. Relax. Relax."*
Sleep restriction – *"Less bedtime for more sleep time."*
Stimulus control – *"Do not multi-task in bed."*
Multi-component cognitive behavioral therapy – *"Let's try everything."*

Mnemonic for Kleine-Levin syndrome: SEXY:
Sleepiness
Eating
Xtacy
Young men

Mnemonic for narcolepsy: CHIPS
Cataplexy
Hallucination
Insomnia (sleep disturbance)
Paralysis
Sleepiness

Therapies for insomnia
Positional therapy for OSA - "Get off your back."
Weight control for obesity and OSA - Fat is bad.
Pharmacologic therapy for OSA: Most don't work.
Mandibular repositioners for OSA: Chin out.
Tongue retainers for OSA: Tongue out.

Upper airway surgery for OSA
What do you call a surgeon who performs the following procedures for OSA:

Nasal septoplasty	*Shape shifter*
Uvulopalatopharyngoplasty	*Palate-thin-ian*
Lingualplasty	*Tongue slasher*
Mandibular advancement	*Jaw breaker*
Tracheotomy	*Cut throat*

Age at which specific EEG features first develop
Sleep spindles: 1 month.
Delta waves: 3 months.
K complexes: 6 months.
 Useful recall tool: 1-3-6 (SO-DO-KU).

Aggregate hours of sleep per day

< 2 months	19	
< 1 year	15	(19 minus 4)
1-3 years	12	(15 minus 3)
3-5 years	10	(12 minus 2)
> 5 years	9	(10 minus 1)

Etiology of sleepiness and fatigue in an adolescent or young adult (8Ds)
Delayed sleep phase disorder (morning sleepiness).
Depression.
Deprivation (sleep).
Disorder (narcolepsy, idiopathic hypersomnia, hypothyroidism, recurrent hypersomnia, obstructive sleep apnea, periodic limb movement disorder) .

Dope (illicit substance).
Drama (malingering).
Drinking.
Drugs (medications).

Insomnia with aging
Men sleep less; women complain more.

Gender difference in prevalence of sleep disorders

Males > females:	SRBD
	RBD
Females > males:	G*IRLS*
	N
	S
	O
	M
	I
	A

Frequency of EEG waves
Order of EEG waves based on increasing Hz: *Do The AlphaBet* or **DTBA** (delta, theta, beta, alpha).

Electrooculography
CO-PO (cornea = positive charge). *RE-NE* (retina = negative charge).
PO-DO-TO (positive voltage = downward deflection = toward an electrode).

General patterns of sleep architecture
High sleep input: ↓ SOL, ↑ SE, ↑ TST and ↓ WASO.
Low sleep input: ↑ SOL, ↓ SE, ↓ TST and ↑ WASO.

Environmental precautions for RBD
"*Protect yourself and others from you.*"

Mnemonic for restless legs syndrome: *IDLE*
Inactivity
Discomfort
Legs
Evening

Alcohol
Alcohol has a biphasic effect on sleep and waking.
Stimulating: At low doses and on the rising phase of alcohol levels. *Note: Visualize an animated person having fun at a bar.*
Sedating: At high doses and on the falling phase of alcohol levels. *Note: Visualize a drowsy person driving home after leaving the bar.*

High school whimsical
There once was a young prince from Istanbul
Who couldn't get up early to go to school
He stayed up all night
But he stood upright when given day light
And majestically declared, "That's cool!"

Phototherapy for jet lag
Get what you do not already have.
You do not need the evening city lights of New York (for eastward travel); instead, get day light.
You do not need the sunny days of California (for westward travel); rather, get evening light.

Fiat lux!
Light exposure *after* CTmin will phase *advance* circadian rhythm.*(Remember: AA: after = advance).*

Circadian rhythm sleep disorders
Irregular sleep-wake disorder: *"Atrial fibrillation" of circadian rhythms (irregularly irregular rhythm).*
Free-running circadian disorder:
> *Three **blind** mice,*
> *three **blind** mice,*
> *see how they "**free run**" ….*

Jet lag: Worse symptoms with eastward travel and aging. *Therefore to minimize symptoms, remember the old adage, "Go west, young man."*

Snoring blues
I don't need no sleep doctor
To tell me that I snore
My wife has told me that before
Now I sleep outside our bedroom door
I need help, sleep doctor, do you have
> *Anything up your sleeve*
To help my poor woman
> *Get some good old-fashioned sleep*
A drug, a pill, a lotion, some magic potion
> *I badly need some me-di-ca-tion.*
Slept on my side, taped my mouth shut
> *Stopped my boozing. I've done all that.*
I'm desperate; I don't want my wife and I to fight
> *So I'll sleep on the living room couch,*
again,

> *tonight.*

Index

Notes

Made in the USA